AF744853

Bacterial Cattle Diseases

Edited by
Hussein Abdel hay El-Sayed Kaoud

Published in London, United Kingdom

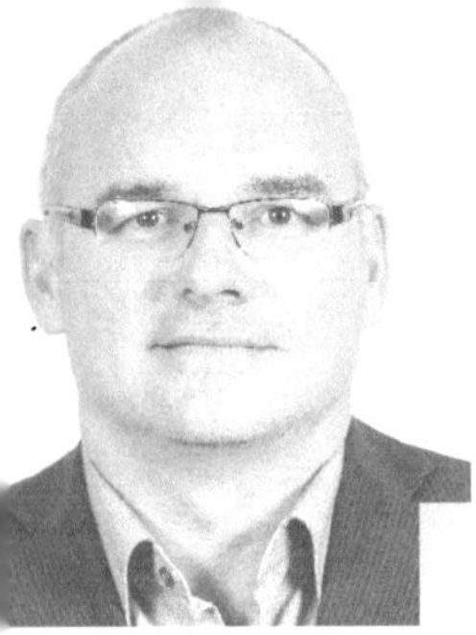
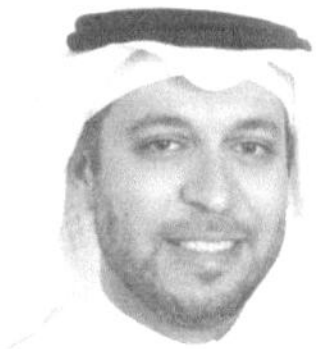
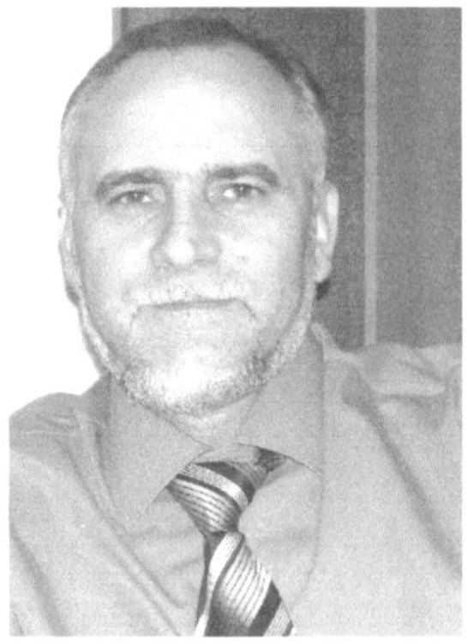
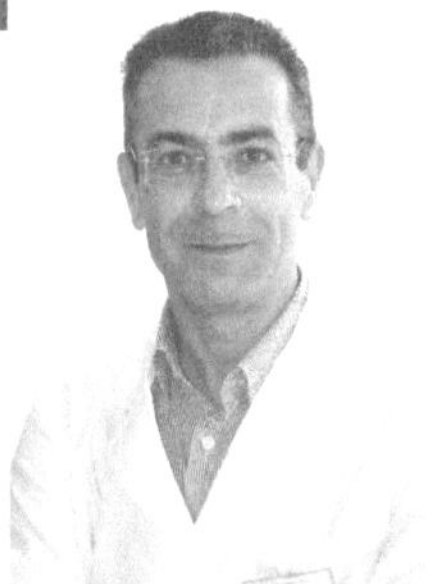
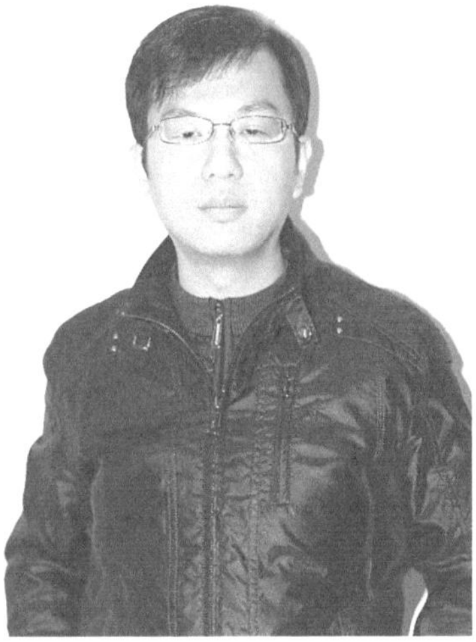
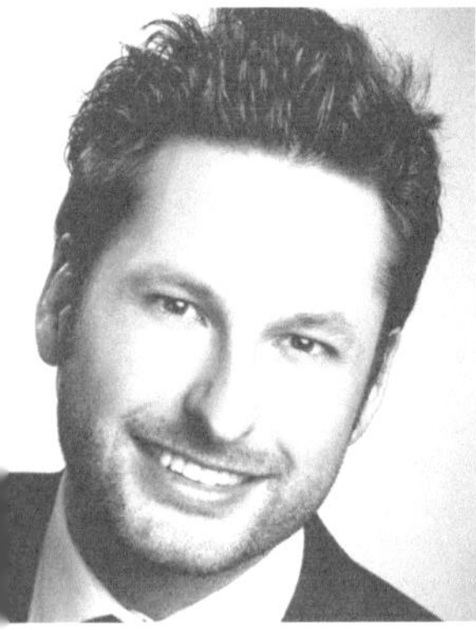
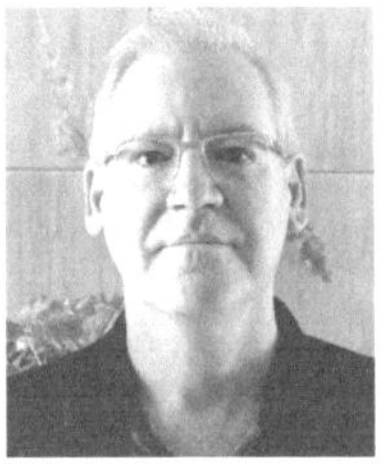

IntechOpen

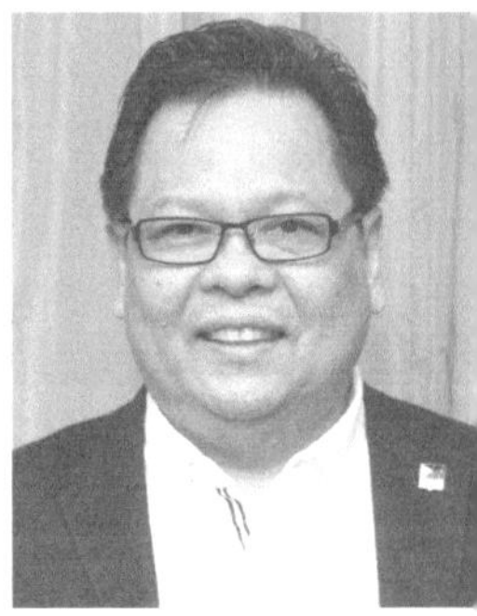
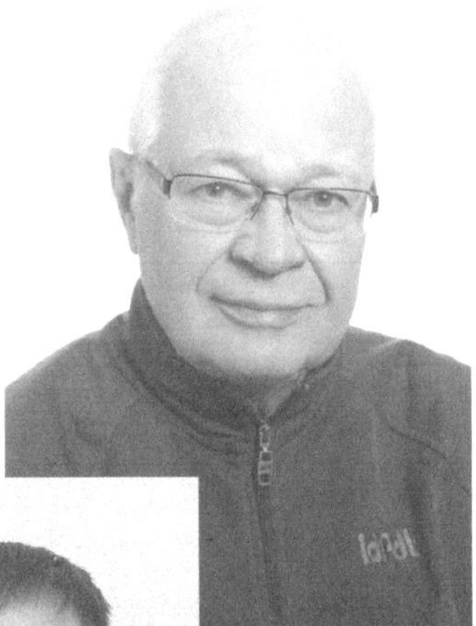
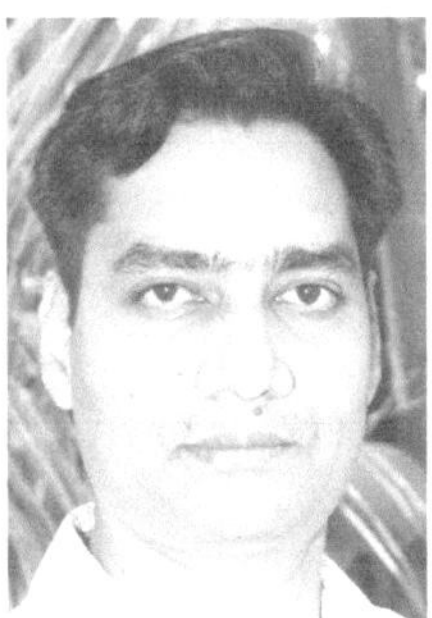
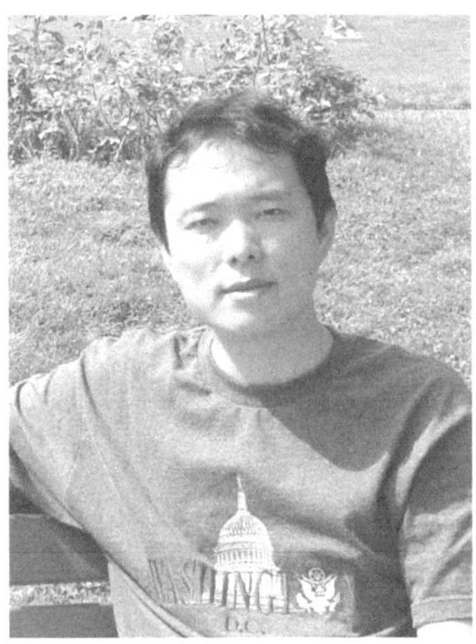
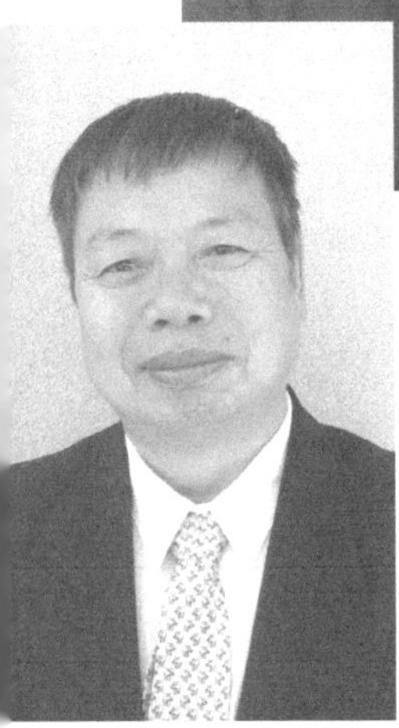
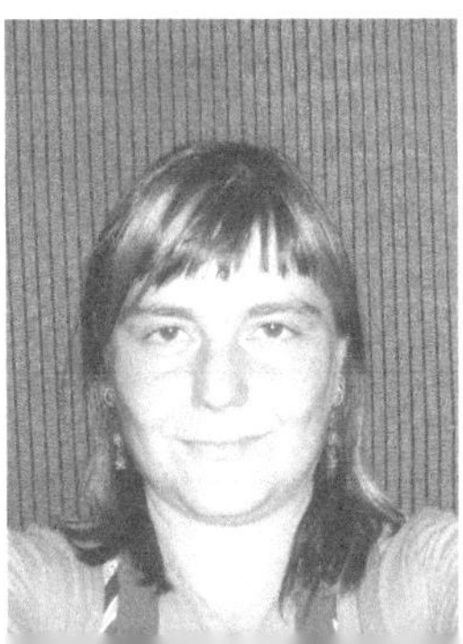

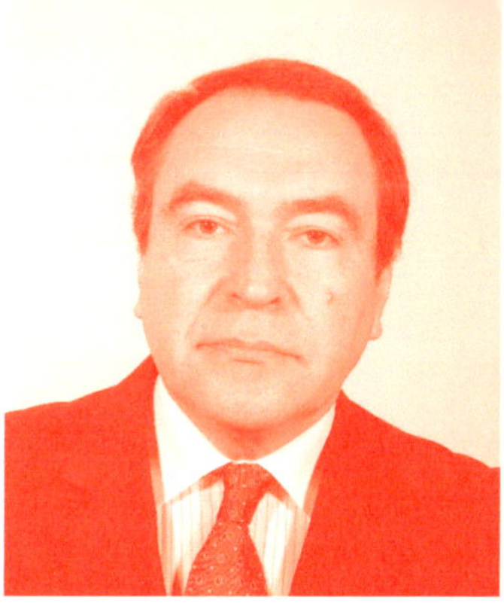

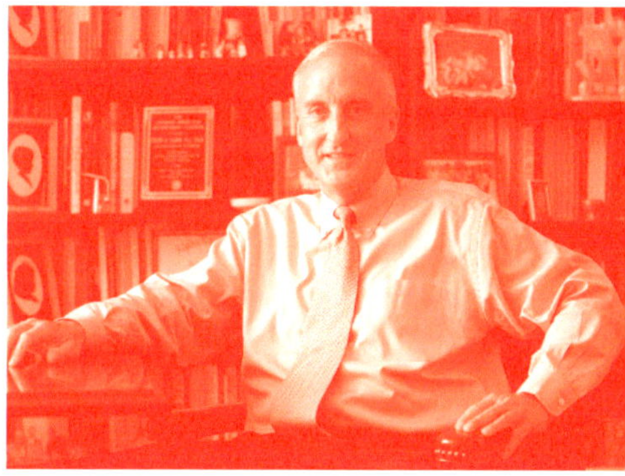

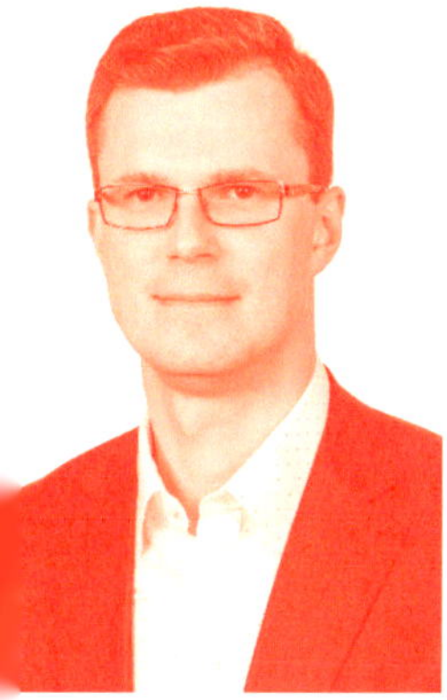

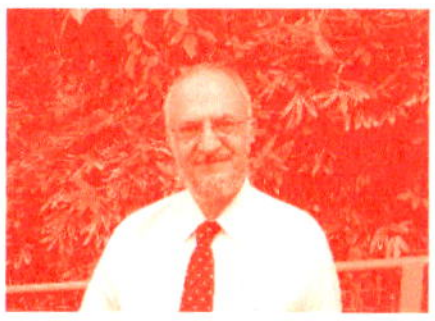

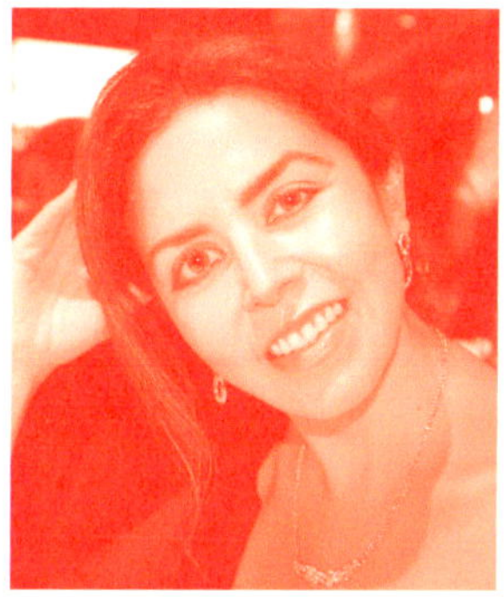

Supporting open minds since 2005

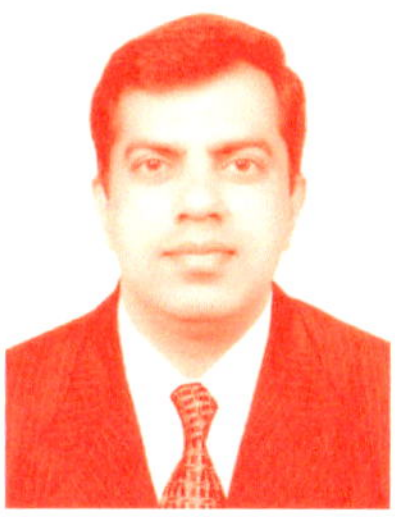

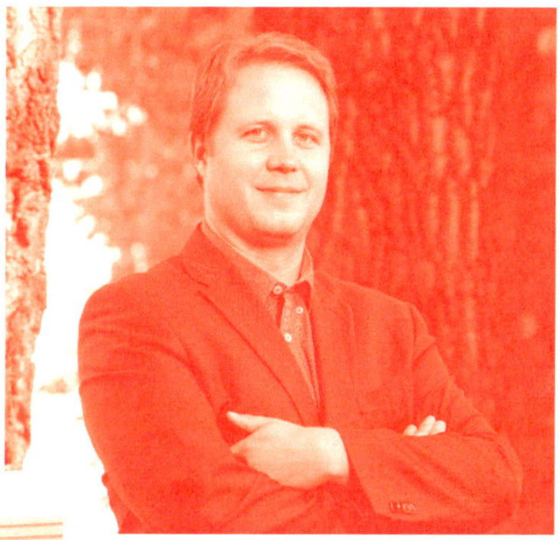

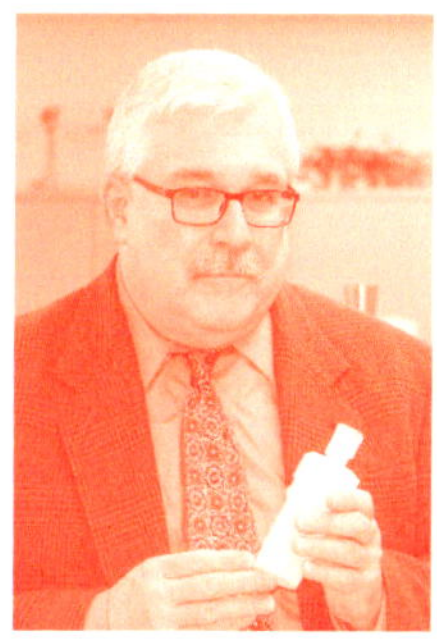

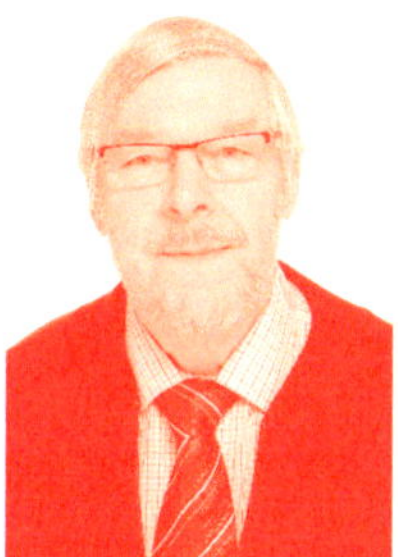

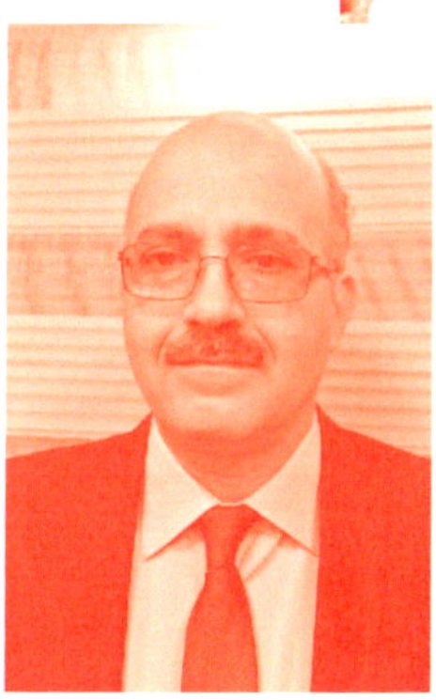

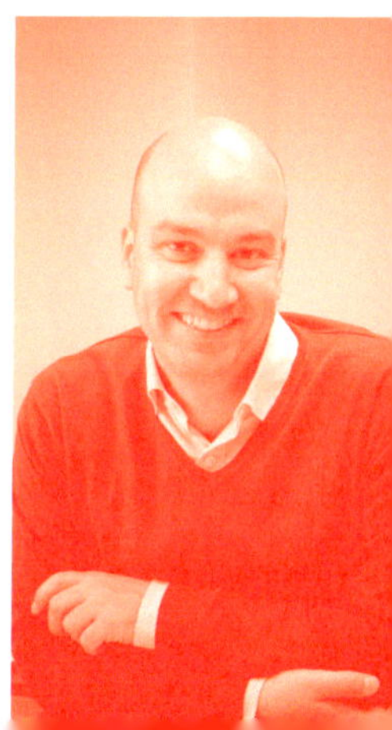

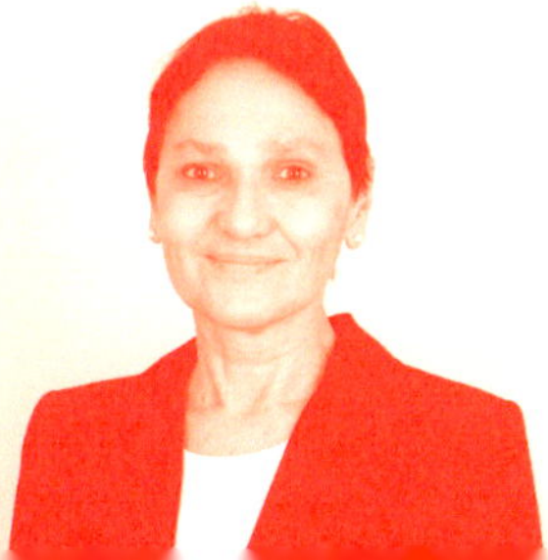

Bacterial Cattle Diseases
http://dx.doi.org/10.5772/intechopen.78416
Edited by Hussein Abdel hay El-Sayed Kaoud

Contributors
Roland Suluku, Jesse Nyandeboh, Sheku Moiforay, Joseph Kuria, Samat Amat, Amjad Islam Aqib, Muhammad Ijaz, Shahid Farooqi, Muhammad Shoaib, Muhammad Alam, Khadija Yasmeen, Hussein Abdelhay Essayed Kaoud

© The Editor(s) and the Author(s) 2019
The rights of the editor(s) and the author(s) have been asserted in accordance with the Copyright, Designs and Patents Act 1988. All rights to the book as a whole are reserved by INTECHOPEN LIMITED. The book as a whole (compilation) cannot be reproduced, distributed or used for commercial or non-commercial purposes without INTECHOPEN LIMITED's written permission. Enquiries concerning the use of the book should be directed to INTECHOPEN LIMITED rights and permissions department (permissions@intechopen.com).
Violations are liable to prosecution under the governing Copyright Law.

Individual chapters of this publication are distributed under the terms of the Creative Commons Attribution 3.0 Unported License which permits commercial use, distribution and reproduction of the individual chapters, provided the original author(s) and source publication are appropriately acknowledged. If so indicated, certain images may not be included under the Creative Commons license. In such cases users will need to obtain permission from the license holder to reproduce the material. More details and guidelines concerning content reuse and adaptation can be found at http://www.intechopen.com/copyright-policy.html.

Notice
Statements and opinions expressed in the chapters are these of the individual contributors and not necessarily those of the editors or publisher. No responsibility is accepted for the accuracy of information contained in the published chapters. The publisher assumes no responsibility for any damage or injury to persons or property arising out of the use of any materials, instructions, methods or ideas contained in the book.

First published in London, United Kingdom, 2019 by IntechOpen
IntechOpen is the global imprint of INTECHOPEN LIMITED, registered in England and Wales, registration number: 11086078, The Shard, 25th floor, 32 London Bridge Street
London, SE19SG – United Kingdom
Printed in Croatia

British Library Cataloguing-in-Publication Data
A catalogue record for this book is available from the British Library

Additional hard and PDF copies can be obtained from orders@intechopen.com

Bacterial Cattle Diseases
Edited by Hussein Abdel hay El-Sayed Kaoud
p. cm.
Print ISBN 978-1-83881-229-4
Online ISBN 978-1-83881-230-0
eBook (PDF) ISBN 978-1-83881-231-7

We are IntechOpen, the world's leading publisher of Open Access books

Built by scientists, for scientists

4,200+
Open access books available

116,000+
International authors and editors

125M+
Downloads

151
Countries delivered to

Our authors are among the

Top 1%
most cited scientists

12.2%
Contributors from top 500 universities

WEB OF SCIENCE™

Selection of our books indexed in the Book Citation Index
in Web of Science™ Core Collection (BKCI)

Interested in publishing with us?
Contact book.department@intechopen.com

Numbers displayed above are based on latest data collected.
For more information visit www.intechopen.com

Meet the editor

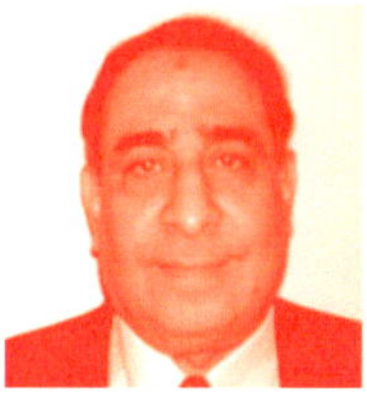

Dr. Hussein Kaoud was the Chairman of the Department of Animal Health and Preventive Medicine at Cairo University. He has attained both a DSc and Veterinary Fellowship. He has given lectures at international universities and has been a member for many of National and International Publishing Houses, and a reviewer and editor for many indexed journals.

Currently, he works as Full Professor at the Faculty of Veterinary Medicine, Cairo University, Egypt. His research interest is focused on molecular biology, molecular epidemiology, and advanced technology of basic life sciences. He has published many publications, and has an international award in the field of Aquaculture (USA), 15 Cairo University International Publication awards, and Appreciation Awards in Advanced Technological Sciences from Cairo University.

Contents

Preface

Cattle constitute one of the major livestock species and are an important economical factor in many countries. The world cattle population is estimated at 1.5 billion animals, more than 1 billion of them in tropical and subtropical countries. They are heavily exposed to numerous bacterial infections, which drastically affect their well-being as well as their productivity. Infectious diseases also play an important economical role in cattle.

This book discusses important bacterial diseases and suggestive prevention strategies based on progress in this field. It includes four sections and five chapters that provide the most common diseases and an overview of the essential methods for their prevention and control.

The book will be useful to researchers and students of veterinary sciences as well as those who are interested in cattle production.

The book is the result of collaborating parties. I gratefully acknowledge the assistance provided by all authors who have contributed to the publication of this volume and the IntechOpen editorial office that initiated this project and saw it to its completion.

The editor is thankful to every individual who helped in the preparation of this book and is also indebted to the chapter contributors for accepting helpful criticism for the present shape of the book.

Finally, thanks are due to Mrs. Marina Dusevic, Author Service Manager of IntechOpen, for sending information and guidelines for editing the book chapters well on time.

Dr. Hussein Abdel hay El-Sayed Kaoud
Full Professor of Preventive Medicine,
Department of Hygiene and Management,
Faculty of Veterinary Medicine,
Cairo University,
El-Giza, Egypt

Section 1

How to Use the Book

Chapter 1

Introductory Chapter: Bacterial Cattle Diseases - Economic Impact and Their Control

Hussien Abdelhay Kaoud

1. Introduction

Many diseases in modern animal farming are thought to have a direct link to the environment with the change of intensive systems with high animal densities on specialized farms; a change in the character of animal diseases took place [1].

Diseases no longer follow the traditional pattern, whereby one specific pathogen provoked clear clinical symptoms with a specific pathology. Intensification also meant that the animal became increasingly dependent on mechanical equipment for mechanical ventilation, feeding, and manure removal.

The considerable increase in herd size and the close contact between animals favor a quick passage of pathogens, which can lead to an increase in virulence and an increased infection pressure [2]. Some animal breeds are productive but may lack sufficient disease resistance and are sensitive to relatively small perturbation in their artificial environment, such as in temperature or air supply.

In contrast to the classical disease of specific etiology, these new disorders are called multifactorial diseases. Multifactorial diseases changed the pattern of diseases, morbidity, and productivity considerably. The characteristic of a multifactorial disease is that there is a variety of internal and external factors involved, and none of the factors alone can produce the disease itself. There are various formulations of the laws of causation, which are applicable to multifactorial infectious and noninfectious diseases [3]. The unified concept of causation by Evans marshals "formal epidemiology" can be applied where a causal hypothesis can be sufficiently probable to provide the rational basis for prophylactic and therapeutic measures. The causation of modem infectious diseases by the relationships between pathogen, host, route of transmission, and environment makes the transition of an infection into a disease possible. The external factors representing the environment include the physical, chemical, and biological environment, housing, management, feed, and water. Together with pathogens or facultative pathogens, these factors influence well-being, health, and performance. A disease, however, will develop only if the "internal factors" of the animal are unable to respond properly. The most important internal factors are genetic disposition (e.g., lack of resistance or adaptation, hormonal dysfunction) and immunity (e.g., maternal antibodies, immunosuppressant).

The aim of this chapter is to inform owners, veterinary professional, and others who are interested in Advanced Veterinary Science dealing with those bacterial infectious diseases, which occur relatively frequently in dairy and beef cattle and focus on general principles for the prevention and control of these diseases, providing detailed information on each disease. The information includes the following: economic impact, recognition of the disease, method of prevention for the spread

IntechOpen

of bacterial diseases between animals in the farm, how to make the animals resist the disease, and the treatment of infected animals.

2. Materials and methods

A *microbial agent* is a microorganism that is capable to cause disease in animal. *Pathogenicity* is the capability to induce disease in an animal. Pathogenic bacteria express their pathological effect by means of their *infectious aggressiveness* (*virulence*), a term which refers to the level of pathogenicity of the microbial organism. Hence, the factors of virulence of a pathogen are any of its genome, biochemical characters, and structure that give the ability to induce disease in an animal. Domestic livestock have always suffered from a wide range of bacterial diseases. As livestock are concentrated in larger numbers, the problems of major epidemic have become more severe.

2.1 Cycle and routes of infection

The epidemiologic triangle (triad model) explains that infectious diseases are produced from the interaction of a causative agent, susceptible animal (host), and environmental surrounding. More attentionally, transmission of the causative agent results when the agent leaves its animal (*host* or *reservoir*) through a way of escape (portal of exit), is produced by some *means of transmission*, and enters through a specific entrance (portal *of entry*) to infect a *susceptible animal*. This cycle is sometimes called the chain of infection.

When speaking of infectious diseases, *exposure* assumes a tailored meaning, namely, encountering the infectious agent in a fashion that allows for agent transmission. Therefore, knowledge of transmission mechanisms is vital for understanding the epidemiology of infectious diseases.

This chapter is focused on major bacterial diseases that can cause significant loss or concern for dairy cattle, beef rearing, and fattening enterprises, as well as practical steps that can be taken to prevent the occurrence of such diseases and regulatory control measures that should be taken on a specific disease.

3. Results and discussion

3.1 *Bovine tuberculosis*

Bovine tuberculosis is a chronic bacterial disease of cattle that sometimes affects other mammalian species. This disease is a major animal disease that can be transmitted to humans, usually by inhaling aerosol or ingestion of unpasteurized milk. The model strategy for the control of diseases in domestic animals includes regular field trials, quarantine, and sanitary wards for infected herds [4]. This prevents the spread of the disease outside the population, while slaughtering infected animals reduces infection from within the farm.

A system of control for the tuberculosis disease in cattle (TB) is by the examination of cattle, which includes slaughtering positive animals (system of test and slaughter) along with the isolation of herds and inducing herd immunization against the disease by vaccination [5]. The health state of the herd is represented by integrating mathematical formulations that express the period of herd quarantine (isolation). The system of TB control in New Zealand can be applied and used as an example (vaccination as control strategy). The induction of such system suggests that vaccine efficacy is more than 95%, reaching 95% of target TB levels within

6 years. These results suggest that the complementary strategy for immunization and vector control may be more promising than vaccination alone [5, 6].

3.2 *Campylobacter enteritis* (Vibrionic enteritis, vibriosis)

Intestinal campylobacteriosis occurs by *Campylobacter jejuni* or *Campylobacter coli*. Although they compete in the digestive system of many species, they can cause diarrhea, especially in small animals. *Campylobacter fetus* can also cause reproductive diseases and abortion in cattle. *Campylobacter* spp., especially *C. jejuni* and *C. coli*, are a major cause of enteritis in humans. Additional species cause venereal diseases in sheep and cattle. Many animals carry *Campylobacter* spp. without any symptoms, throwing the organism in their feces or stools. Bulls can be vaccinated annually against the campylobacteriosis [5].

Vaccinations are also available for cows and make the animal very resistant to infection. It can help biosecurity and the examination of bulls purchased in the identification of the disease. If the ox has to be bought, the best policy is the younger the better. If you are forced to buy a mature bull, use antibiotics before using it to breed cows and use them on a small number of cows only so that their fertility can be recorded before they are used for service in the original herd.

3.3 Anthrax

Anthrax is caused by *Bacillus anthracis*, a spore and a gram-positive rod in the Bacillaceae family. The anthrax is completely malignant with plasmid pX01, which denotes the trioxide complex of the protein, and pX02, which encodes the capsule genes. *B. anthracis* is very homogenous genetically. However, researchers identified several genetically distinct groups that appear to be derived from cloned animals. Some of these clones are distributed worldwide, while others are in limited geographical areas [1, 5].

Infection is usually acquired through the ingestion of contaminated soil, feed, or mixed fodder. Anthrax spores in soil are very resistant and can cause disease when ingested even after years of outbreaks, the spores are brought to the surface due to wet weather or by deep tillage. When the disease appears or is inhaled by ruminants, the disease appears. In the event of an outbreak, the bodies of succumbed animals should be buried or burned properly and the carcass or body forbidden be open (because exposure to air results in forming spores). The buildings, region, or houses should be put under quarantine until all susceptible animals are vaccinated.

A prophylactic measure by vaccination in endemic areas is utmost significant. In spite of vaccination seeming to prevent outbreaks, veterinary authorities may forget to vaccinate susceptible animals when the disease does not occur for several years (spores of the anthrax stay alive for long intervals), so the risk is always present. Anthrax disease is recorded in the list of the World Health Organization (WHO), Animal Health Code (OIE), 2011, (Article 1.2.3) and must be reported to the OIE (Chapter 1.1.2—Disease Notification and Epidemiological Information).

4. Bacterial respiratory affections

4.1 Hemorrhagic septicemia

The disease results from certain serotypes of *Pasteurella multocida*, a gram-negative coccobacillus, which is often used as a nasopharyngeal animal. The Asian cultivar B:2 and the African serotype E:2 (Carter and Heddleston classification), corresponding to the classification of 6:B and 6:E (Namioka-Carter), are the two main culprits. A:1 and A:3 have been associated with a condition similar to HS in cattle and buffaloes in India with pneumonia in the first place leading to death. The letter refers to the antigen of the wallet and indicates the number of physical antigens [1, 3].

4.2 Contagious bovine pleuropneumonia

Caused by *Mycoplasma mycoides* subsp. *Mycoides* (the bovine biotype). *Mycoplasma mycoides* are a small colony type, belonging to the *Mycoplasmataceae* family. It can be categorized into two major lineages [1–3]:

1. Isolates from Europe

2. Isolates from Africa

Other strains of *M. mycoides* were retrieved from other animal species (goats or sheep). The other strains are similar antigenically to bovine strains; they do not appear to be pathogenic to cattle, but they may cause diseases other than CBPP in small ruminants.

4.3 *Mannheimia haemolytica*

Serotype 1 of *Mannheimia haemolytica* is the common isolated bacteria of the cow's respiratory tract with BRD. *Pasteurella multocida* is also an important reason of pneumonia. *Histophilus somni* is constantly recognized as an important pathogen in bacterial respiratory disease (BRD). These bacteria are normal inhabitants of the nasal pharynx of cattle. When pulmonary abscess occurs, it is generally associated with chronic pneumonia.

4.4 *Trueperella pyogenes*

Trueperella pyogenes is frequently isolated in bacterial respiratory disease (BRD).

4.5 Chronic suppurative pulmonary disease

Chronic lung suppurative disease develops due to unsuccessful treatment or incomplete recovery from previous lung attacks. The outbreak of bacterial infection in the lungs is often associated with a stressful event such as transport, sale, or the most common. Salmonellosis, especially *Salmonella* infection (*Salmonella Dublin* infection), and Johne's disease are other examples of postnatal reinfection.

4.6 *Mycoplasma pneumoniae*

Mycoplasma bovis is one of the emerging causes of respiratory diseases and arthritis in cows and in dairy calves and fattening calves. Experimental infection usually leads to a lack of access to mild signs of respiratory disease, but malignant strains that cause severe lung disease have been identified in calves [5].

1. The greatest risk is the purchase of cattle or calves, clinically or subclinically infected with *Mycoplasma bovis*.

2. Maintaining a completely closed herd policy is the best way to reduce the risk of introducing *Mycoplasma bovis*.

3. If you have to buy cows or heifers, there is always the risk of buying the infection. This risk can be minimized through a detailed history, only the purchase of herds of few somatic cells, and by examining the herd from which the animals were purchased, or individuals who were quarantined before entering the main herd, by means of serum tests.

4. Feeding milk waste is not recommended to calves where *Mycoplasma bovis* has been diagnosed.

5. Although there are no commercial vaccines licensed in Europe for *Mycoplasma bovis*, APHA and other companies are licensed to produce a self-produced vaccine.

5. Control of bacterial respiratory affections

The pathological mechanism includes environmental and management pressures and perhaps an initial viral infection followed by secondary bacterial infection in the lower respiratory tract. Stress results from environmental and husbandry factors, including inadequate ventilation, mixing with the addition of calves to a specific group, overcrowding, and feeding practices such as poor quality milk replacer. Failure of the negative transmission of mother immunity (maternal antibodies) is a critical factor for the appearance and induction of the disease [7].

Mycoplasma mycoides, *Pasteurella multocida*, *Mannheimia haemolytica*, *and Mycoplasma bovis* are the most causes *of bacterial respiratory affections*. The risk and degree of pneumonia can be ameliorated by good managemental practices, adequate housing, and adequate ventilation, good breeding, and good nursing care. Control starts by immunization of mothers (vaccinating cows) against certain respiratory pathogens at 3–4 weeks before calving to produce good quality of the antibodies in colostrums. Newly born calves should receive good quality of colostrums of 8–10% body weights in the first 6 hours after parturition. Newborn calves should be individually placed in adequate houses and consumed whole milk or high-quality milk substitutes with a fiber content less than 0.25% for a period of 8–12 weeks of age.

Prophylactic measures should be taken such as:

- Long-acting antibiotics should be given upon arrival of animals after transportation of cattle in the farms.

- Prophylaxis has been shown to significantly:

  a. reduce morbidity;

  b. improve gain; and

  c. add medicaments in ration or drinking water that have limited value because oral antibiotics are poorly absorbed in ruminants.

5.1 Bovine brucellosis

Bovine brucellosis, caused by *Brucella abortus* bacteria, is an economically important cause of abortion in cows. Abortion also affects other species, including bison, buffalo, and elk; some species are host maintenance for this organism. Infection in the wild animals can hinder efforts to eradicate the disease in bovine. In the same time, *B. abortus* transmitted to humans (zoonotic disease). In humans, brucellosis causes debilitating and sometimes chronic disease that affects different organs. Many cases are the result from the contact with infected animals but also occur from ingestion of contaminated food [5, 8].

In low-prevalence conditions, control of *bovine brucellosis* (BB) can be achieved by combining test and slaughter programs with stringent biosecurity measures and removing of reactors. However, in high-incidence cases, immunization can help the control of outbreaks that reduce the rate of infection at both individual and herd levels.

Vaccination with RB51 permits a rapid reduction in the susceptible herds and flocks in an endemic regions, resulting in a rapid decline in the incidence of disease from occurring; this, combined with the frequent testing, permitted the control and eradication of the disease after 3–5 years.

A combination of strict biosecurity measures, strong diagnostic pressure, and vaccination program is able to reduce the spread of BB. The RB51 vaccination allows rapid reduction in vulnerable populations in a highly contagious environment, contributing to a rapid decline in individual infection; this, together with repeated testing, allowed control and eventual elimination after 3–5 years

5.2 Listeriosis

Listeriosis is an infectious disease caused by bacteria, *Listeria monocytogenes*. It is an animal disease. Listeriosis is primarily the winter sickness of the winter feedlot or ruminant dwells. The less acidic pH of the corroded silage enhances the multiplication of *L. monocytogenes*. Listeriosis occurs intermittently in cows, where most cases are associated with feeding fermented and poorly preserved feeds. Listeriosis is an infectious but not contagious disease caused by *Listeria monocytogenes*, which is more common in domestic animals (mammals and domestic poultry), especially ruminants, than humans and is sporadic but can occur like an outbreak in ruminant farms. Listeriosis is treated with antibiotics, depending on the shape of the disease; treatment may take up to 6 weeks or more [5].

High doses are required because of the difficulty in achieving minimum concentrations of antibiotics in the brain. Recovery depends on early and aggressive antibiotics. If signs of encephalitis are severe, death usually occurs despite treatment. The risk of listeriosis can be reduced by feeding good quality silage with low pH. Avoid the bad or decomposed silage or the high-grade silage (a few inches) that have been exposed to air. Any remaining residual fodder should be removed at no cost after feeding. Anti-rodents will prevent the spread of bacteria. Vaccines are available in some countries, but the results are questionable, leading to questions about the cost-benefit of vaccination.

5.3 Leptospirosis

Leptospirosis is a bacterial infection that has identified five common serovars causing abortion in cattle: *Leptospira canicola*, *L. icterohaemorrhagiae*, *L. grippotyphosa*, *L. hardjo*, and *L. pomona*. Leptospirosis is spread by infected urine or contaminated water (by mice). Control of *Leptospira hardjo* in herds depends on a range of management decisions to reduce the risk of infection, strategic treatment with antibiotics, and vaccination. The main pathway to immunization consists of two spaced injections of 4 weeks followed by an annual lift. Vaccination should prevent the execration of the microorganism in urine after exposure and protect against falling milk and abortion.

In contaminated regions, herds without previous infection of leptospiroses, all animals of the herd, including bulls, should be quarantined and isolated for 21 days and given 25 mg/kg streptomycin two times for 10–14 days interval before entering the herd. Herds of acute leptospiroses infection should be under a comprehensive antibiotic treatment to reduce the risk of infection and immunization. Herds in an endemic regions should be vaccinated annually. Replacement heifers should have completed their vaccination course before first service. As a precautionary measure, streptomycin is added to the semen from bulls held at artificial insemination centers.

5.4 Clostridial diseases

These include blackleg disease, malignant edema, black disease, enterotoxemia, and redwater disease. All these diseases are common. The organisms form spores that can live for long periods in hostile environments and kill cattle quickly, giving little chance of treatment. Clostridial organisms are mostly normal flora of cattle and become only a problem with food stress, injury, management changes, parasitism, or other unusual conditions that create a favorable growth environment and produce strong toxins. While some diseases rarely occur, most of them occur sporadically in herds. Clostridium disease has generally very poor prognosis, and the first sign of the disease may be death. Because treatment success is rare, proper emphasis is placed on preventive measures [1–3].

Vaccines are widely used in the dairy industry and can be an effective way to reduce losses due to these bacteria. Single vaccination with most clostridial vaccines does not provide adequate levels of protection and should be followed with a booster dose within 3–6 weeks after the first one. Vaccination of calves gives protective immunity for 1–2 months, so the adequate immunization for calves is obtained through vaccination of the pregnant cows, so that maximum immunity and protection are transferred to the calves in the colostrums. Inactivated vaccines, including 2–8 of clostridium types, should be taken at the age of susceptibility to provide maximum and efficient protection.

Livestock diseases cost farmers millions of pounds a year. In addition to deaths, loss of production and loss of animal wealth often(succumbed). Unsolicited animals require more food and take longer to grow than health stocks. The good animal health program calls for full operation between owner and veterinarians. Farmers must also know that many of the diseases that live in stocks go from animal to animal to human. Animals usually acquire diseases either by (1) contact with diseased animals or (2) improper sanitation, nutrition, care, and management.

Protecting the health of animals by restricting purchases to healthy flocks through appropriate quarantine when bringing in new animals through the use of sound sanitation, management, and nutrition principles and using appropriate and reliable vaccines and vaccines for disease prevention is an economic way to avoid disease losses. Prevention of diseases is better and more economical than rushing to control disease outbreaks.

There are three kinds of control measures [1]:

1. *reducing or eliminating the source or reservoir of infection*: (isolation, quarantine, and therapy for elimination of bacterial infections via antibiotics and destruction of an animal reservoir of infection via laboratory tests, environmental control, and sanitation);

2. *breaking the connection between the source of the infection and susceptible animals* via disinfection and sanitation; and

3. *reducing the number of susceptible animals* by mass immunization.

Immunization can be divided into:

- *passive immunization* which provides temporary immunity after exposure to a pathogen or when a disease threatens to take epidemic pattern; and
- *active immunization* which protects animals from pathogens and populations. During the production of antibodies after effective immunization against the disease, there is often an increase in exposure to the disease in question. The period in which immunity varies from vaccine to vaccine. For a given disease, a second booster dose is required after the first vaccination to achieve stronger immunity. Vaccination can be used proactively to give protection but no substitute for good sanitation.

Some vaccines are highly effective:

- *Campylobacter fetus* vaccine (oil adjuvant vaccine);
- entire *Pasteurella* whole cell bacterins (free of leucotoxoids to avoid the severity of bovine respiratory disease); and
- clostridium toxoids vaccines: *Clostridium chauvoei* (blackleg) and *Clostridium septicum* (malignant edema) are highly effective.

Although the vaccine has improved the situation, it certainly did not prevent the problem. Other control measures, such as rigorous testing of small bulls and the execution or culling of older bulls and late cows, may be more economically beneficial. Some vaccines such as leptospirosis are more effective against nonhost modified strains of host-adapted strains. The general rule is that if postpartum infection leads to a chronic pregnant animal, which means that the animal's immune system has not been able to eliminate the infection, the development of a vaccine that stimulates the immune system adequately to prevent infection is difficult if not impossible. Therefore, the general view is that vaccines can reduce the rate of morbidity (the number of infected animals) and reduce the rate of mortality (deaths) of clinical cases. On the other hand, vaccination alone will not completely prevent the problem and may be other measures of control is equal or more important.

Biosecurity reduces the introduction or the incidence of disease in farms, reduces the spread of diseases already found on farms, and reduces the risk of disease transmission among farms. Biosecurity controls the transmission of pathogens among animals, from animals to fodder, and animals to equipment that may relate directly or indirectly to other animals. Biosecurity practices prevent the spread of disease by reducing the movement of biological organisms and their vectors (viruses, bacteria, rodents, pesticides, etc.) into and within operations through animals, vehicles, visitors, employees, pests, and other means. While the development and maintenance of biosecurity is difficult, it is the cheapest and most effective means of controlling disease, and the disease prevention program will not work without it.

Measures for the prevention and control of disease-producing agents:

- Avoid the introduction of causative agents to the farm or the herd (maintain a closed herd)

The first step is to avoid purchasing cattle from unknown source or purchase from healthy herds.

Owners would have to strictly adhere to the following requirements:

- use homegrown replacements for maintaining and increasing herd size;
- prevent contacts of stock with other cattle herds;
- use artificial insemination for breeding;
- avoid exhibits or shows; and
- apply restricted measures against visitors.
- Quarantine measures

Isolate new arrivals or the purchased animals and apply the following measures:

- separate housing, feeding, and calving areas;
- prevent contact with other animals;
- prevent manure movement from the isolation area to the rest of the herd;
- quarantine or isolated period is 21–30 days; and
- observe and examine for early disease detection.
- Use laboratory testing before purchasing animals

Owners should take precautions when purchasing animals and use laboratory-testing programs to prevent the introduction of diseases to their animals, so the following precautions should be taken:

- purchase disease-free pregnant or virgin heifers to minimize the risk of introducing mastitis;
- vaccinate the purchased animals if necessary according to the vaccinal program of the farm;
- purchase animals from healthy and certified herd under the health accredited herds program; and
- the purchased animals must be guaranteed or *isolated for 21–30 days for*:
    1. Bacterial culture of milk
    2. Blood testing for specific diseases
- Use vaccines

Vaccines are commonly used to protect cattle against respiratory disease and abortion. For herd additions, these vaccines may be given during the 21- to 30-day isolation period. Vaccination against the diseases should be the cornerstone of every herd vaccination program. Consult your veterinarian for specific recommendations on these and other aspects of health management for livestock.

6. Conclusion

Livestock diseases cost farmers millions of pounds a year. In addition to deaths, loss of production and loss of animal wealth often. Farmers must also know that many of the diseases that live in stocks go from animal to animal to human. Animals usually acquire diseases either by (1) contact with diseased animals or (2) improper sanitation, nutrition, care, and management.

Protecting the health of animals by restricting purchases to healthy flocks through appropriate quarantine when bringing in new animals through the use of sound sanitation, management, and nutrition principles and using appropriate and reliable vaccines and vaccines for disease prevention is an economic way to avoid disease losses. Prevention of diseases is better and more economical than rushing to control disease outbreaks.

Author details

Hussien Abdelhay Kaoud
Full Professor of Animal, Poultry, Aquaculture Health and Environmental Pollution, Department of Veterinary Hygiene and Management, Faculty of Veterinary Medicine, Cairo University, El-Giza, Egypt

*Address all correspondence to: ka-oud@link.net

IntechOpen

© 2019 The Author(s). Licensee IntechOpen. This chapter is distributed under the terms of the Creative Commons Attribution License (http://creativecommons.org/licenses/by/3.0), which permits unrestricted use, distribution, and reproduction in any medium, provided the original work is properly cited.

References

[1] Kaoud HA. Cattle Health Diseases, Prevention and Control, Management, Husbandry and Production. Copyright© 2000-2015, CreateSpace, North Charleston- US: A DBA Publishing, LLC; 2015. pp. 79-110

[2] Kaoud HA. Principals of Veterinary Epidemiology. Copyright© 2000-2015, CreateSpace; North Charleston- US: A DBA Publishing, LLC; 2015. pp. 208-213

[3] Kaoud HA. Biosecurity (Health Protection and Sanitation STrategies). In: Animal Farms. Copyright© 2000-2015, CreateSpace; North Charleston- US: A DBA Publishing, LLC; 2015. pp. 178-181

[4] Michigan Bovine Tuberculosis Eradication Project. Available from: http://www.michigan.gov/emergingdiseases/0,1607,7-186-25804-74719--,00.html

[5] World Organization for Animal Health (OIE). http://www.oie.int. OIE Manual of Diagnostic Tests and Vaccines for Terrestrial Animals. Available from: http://www.oie.int/international-standard-setting/terrestrial-manual/access-online

[6] Pollock JM, Rodgers JD, Welsh MD, McNair J. Pathogenesis of bovine tuberculosis: The role of experimental models of infection. Veterinary Microbiology. 2006;**112**:141-150

[7] Centers for Disease Control and Prevention [CDC]. Brucellosis (*Brucella melitensis*, *abortus*, *suis*, and *canis*). CDC; 2005 Oct. Available from: http://www.cdc.gov/ncidod/dbmd/diseaseinfo/brucellosis_t.htm

[8] Borriello G, Capparelli R, Bianco M, Fenizia D, Alfano F, Capuano F, et al. Genetic resistance to *Brucella abortus* in the water buffalo (*Bubalus bubalis*). Infection and Immunity. 2006;**74**:2115-2120

Section 2

Problem of Respiratory Diseases in Cattle

Chapter 2

Bovine Respiratory Disease in Feedlot Cattle: Antimicrobial Resistance in Bovine Respiratory Bacterial Pathogens and Alternative Antimicrobial Approaches

Samat Amat

Abstract

Bovine respiratory disease (BRD) is the leading cause of morbidity and mortality in feedlot cattle in North America. The BRD is a complex multifactorial disease because its onset depends on the interaction between number of factors including host, environment, management and viral and bacterial infectious agents. The main bacterial pathogens associated with BRD are *Mannheimia haemolytica, Pasteurella multocida, Histophilus somni* and *Mycoplasma bovis.* Treatment and prevention of BRD in the feedlots are aimed mainly at bacterial pathogens through antimicrobial use. Although antimicrobial use has increased, the prevalence of BRD has also increased potentially due to the emergence of multidrug-resistant bacterial pathogens, which poses a serious threat to both animal and public health and necessitates the development of alternative antimicrobial approaches to mitigate BRD pathogens in feedlot cattle. The objective of this chapter is to provide a brief overview of pathogenesis of BRD, to review the current status of antimicrobial resistance in bacterial pathogens associated with BRD, and to discuss the potential antimicrobial alternative strategies, including probiotic and essential oil (EO) approaches, to mitigate bovine respiratory pathogens in feedlot cattle.

Keywords: bovine respiratory disease, bacterial pathogens, antimicrobial resistance, antimicrobial alternatives, feedlot cattle

1. Introduction

Cattle production is one of the important industries in North America, accounting for $78.2 billion (US) and $10.5 billion (Canada) in cash receipts during 2015. A substantial part of this economic benefit is derived from beef sector, where 10.6 and 2.5 million head of cattle and calves in the USA and Canada, respectively, were slaughtered for the beef market in 2015 [1, 2]. The number of beef cattle in the North American farms and ranches will continue to increase over the next decade due to the growing red meat demand by an increasing world population, with an estimated increase from 7.6 billion people in 2017 to 8.6 billion people in 2030 [3].

Despite advances in veterinary medicine, animal husbandry and animal welfare, economic impacts of cattle disease on the beef cattle industry still remain significant, with BRD being the most significant health problem in modern feedlot industry in North America. Bovine respiratory disease is commonly associated with pneumonia in nursing beef calves and recently weaned feedlot cattle. Cattle are mostly affected by BRD within the first 45 days after feedlot placement [4, 5]. According to the Feedlot 2011 study conducted by the National Animal Health Monitoring System (NAHMS), 97% of feedlots across the USA reported having cattle with BRD, and 16.2% of the cattle in a feedlot were affected by BRD during the feeding period [6]. The annual financial loss attributed to BRD, including mortality, reduced feed efficiency and performance and treatment costs, has been estimated to be more than $4 billion to the US beef industry [7]. This loss surpasses the economic losses incurred by all other cattle diseases combined [8], given that BRD accounts for 70–80% of all morbidity and 40–50% of all mortality in the US feedlots [9].

Bovine respiratory disease is a complex disease with a multitude of stressors that predispose cattle to viral and bacterial infection. *Mannheimia haemolytica*, *Pasteurella multocida*, *Histophilus somni* and *Mycoplasma bovis* are the main bacterial pathogens involved in BRD and are, therefore, the main targets of antimicrobial treatments to control BRD [10]. In the North American feedlots, cattle considered at high risk for the development of clinical BRD signs are often given antimicrobial metaphylaxis upon feedlot arrival to prevent BRD [11]. However, recent studies have shown the emergence of BRD bacterial pathogens that are resistant to several classes of antibiotics used to both control and treat BRD [12–14]. The multidrug resistance in BRD pathogens towards particularly tilmicosin, tulathromycin and oxytetracycline has been increased in feedlot cattle in the last decade [15], and such increase may partially due to the increased use of these antibiotics as metaphylaxis. The continued rise in AMR in BRD bacterial pathogens necessitates the developing antimicrobial alternative approaches to mitigate bacterial pathogens associated with BRD in feedlot cattle. Recent research results suggest the potential use of probiotic and essential oil (EO) as antibiotic alternative approaches to mitigate bovine respiratory pathogens [16, 17]. The objective of this chapter is to provide a brief overview of pathogenesis of BRD, to review the current status of antimicrobial resistance in bacterial pathogens associated with BRD and to discuss the potential antimicrobial alternative strategies, including probiotic and EO approaches, to mitigate bovine respiratory pathogens in feedlot cattle.

2. Bovine respiratory disease (BRD)

2.1 Pathogenesis of BRD

2.1.1 Predisposing factors

Bovine respiratory disease, also known as a shipping fever, is a complex multifactorial disease because its onset depends on the interaction between number of factors including host, environment, management and viral and bacterial infectious agents (**Figure 1**) [18]. The host factors predisposing cattle to BRD include age, body weight, immune status and genetics [18]. The age and body weight of the calves entering the feedlot are, in most cases, inversely correlated with disease

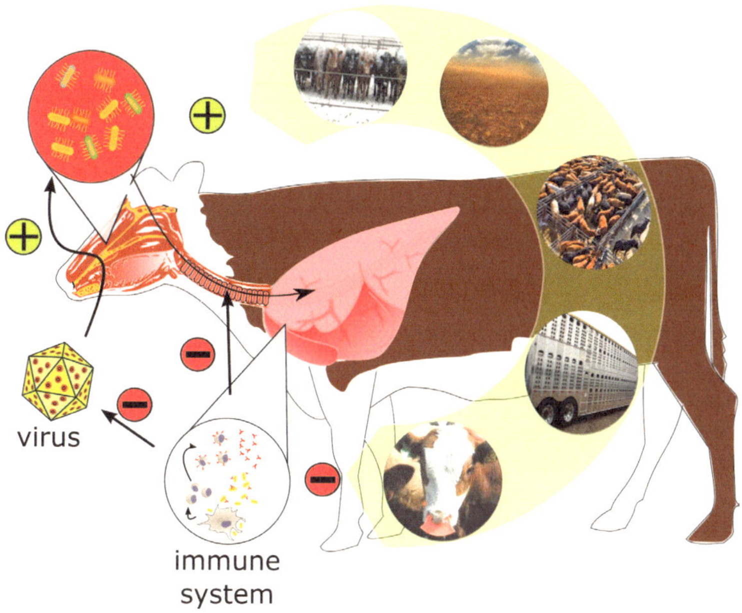

Figure 1.
Schematic overview of the pathogenesis of bovine respiratory disease in cattle.

susceptibility to BRD during the feeding phase [19, 20]. Shipping is the leading environmental risk factor for BRD due to the fact that almost all cattle placed in the feedlot are transported from elsewhere. Transportation distance has a negative impact on the animal resistance to the development of BRD owing to the stress and body weight loss that occur during the transportation [18]. In addition, commingling with other cattle in sale barns is an important management factor predisposing cattle to BRD. Because sale barn cattle have greater exposure to pathogens and stress as a result of mixing with cattle from multiple sources, feedlot cattle purchased from sale barn are often at greater risk for BRD compared to the ones purchased directly from the farm or ranch. Of note, the host, environment and management factors discussed above are necessary but not always sufficient to cause pneumonia, and thus, additional predisposing factors, such as viral infection, are often necessary to produce bacterial pneumonia [18].

2.1.2 Viral agents

The most common viral agents associated with BRD include bovine herpesvirus type 1 (BHV-1), parainfluenza-3 virus (PI3), bovine viral diarrhea virus (BVDV) and bovine respiratory syncytial virus (BRSV) [13]. These viral pathogens can induce primary infection with mild clinical signs of BRD and predispose cattle to bacterial infection [18, 21]. Viral infection can impair the mucosal barrier and respiratory pathogen clearance, damage the lung parenchyma and suppress immune responses in cattle. Combined, the effects of viral infection facilitate the proliferation of opportunistic bacterial pathogens in the upper respiratory tract and translocation of these pathogens into the lung and cause infections to the compromised lung [21]. A recent human study suggested that respiratory viruses can also affect the structure and composition of nasal microbiota, which may be another way through which virus weakens host resistance to bacterial pathogens [22].

2.1.3 Bacterial agents

The main bacterial pathogens associated with BRD are *M. haemolytica, P. multocida, H. somni* and *M. bovis* [10]. *M. haemolytica* is the principal bacterial agent of BRD and has a considerable economic impact on the North American feedlot industry. It is a small, Gram-negative and facultative anaerobic bacterium that commonly exists as a part of nasopharyngeal and tonsillar crypt microbiota in healthy cattle and sheep [23]. To date, 12 different (1, 2, 5–9, 12–14 and 16–17) capsular serotypes have been identified within *M. haemolytica* [23]. Among these serotypes, serotype 1 (S1), serotype 2 (S2) and serotype 6 (S6) are most frequently isolated from feedlot cattle, with the S1 and S6 being the most prevalent in bovine infection [24, 25]. *M. haemolytica* residing in the upper respiratory tract of healthy cattle maintains a commensal relationship with the host due to the containment by the local microbiota and host immunity [23]. However, when the local microbiota and host immunity get disrupted by stress and viral infections, this opportunistic bacterium proliferates in the upper respiratory tract and then translocates into the lung where it induces acute infection characteristics to fibrinous pneumonia [23]. *M. haemolytica*-induced pathogenesis is accomplished through a combination of virulence factors including outer membrane proteins, leukotoxin (Lkt), lipopolysaccharide (LPS) and lipoproteins [23]. The outer membrane proteins, such as adhesion protein, facilitate attachment and colonization of *M. haemolytica* to the bovine respiratory cells. The Lkt, being the most important virulence factor, attracts neutrophils and macrophages to the site of infection when it is present in low concentration. High levels of Lkt, however, induce cell death of leukocytes and phagocytes, allowing *M. haemolytica* to evade the detection and destruction by the host immune system. The other virulent factors, including LPS and lipoproteins, are involved in hemorrhage, edema, hypoxemia and acute inflammation [10]. The virulence factors of *M. haemolytica* differ among different serotypes, and such difference has been reported to attribute to the genetic differences among serotypes [25].

P. multocida and *H. somni* are also opportunistic BRD pathogens and are involved in the development of bronchopneumonia in cattle with clinical signs indistinguishable from pneumonia caused by *M. haemolytica*. The isolation rate of *P. multocida* and *H. somni* from clinically healthy cattle at feedlot entry is relatively high ranging from 15% up to 60% [10], suggesting they predominately exist as part of normal nasopharyngeal flora in healthy cattle. However, the isolation rate of these two pathogens is higher in the lower respiratory tract of feedlot cattle affected by BRD compared to healthy cattle [13]. The main virulence factors identified in *P. multocida* include a LPS, a cytotoxin, and iron acquisition proteins [10]. *H. somni* virulence factors include expression of immunoglobulin-binding proteins, survival in phagocytic cells, induction of apoptosis in endothelial cells, antigenic phase variation and endotoxic activity of the LPS and biofilm formation [10].

Compared to the other three BRD bacterial pathogens, *M. bovis* is the least characterized BRD pathogen. This bacterium lacks a cell wall and is fastidious, requiring specialized media and techniques for its isolation and culture. *M. bovis* is often associated with chronic pneumonia, and its mechanism of actions remains poorly understood [10].

2.2 Current prevention and control strategies for BRD in feedlots

Prevention and control of BRD in large commercial feedlots in North America are aimed mainly at bacterial pathogens, through the use of antimicrobials and vaccination programs. Cattle considered at high risk for the development of BRD are often given metaphylactic antimicrobials upon feedlot arrival [26]. Metaphylaxis is defined as the mass treatment of an entire group or population of cattle with an antimicrobial to prevent and minimize an expected outbreak of disease [26]. Overall, 59.3% of feedlots in the USA with a capacity of >1000 head cattle use injective metaphylaxis, with approximately 21.3% of the cattle placed in the feedlot, receive metaphylactic antibiotics [6]. In Western Canada, more than 80% of the cattle in some feedlots receive injectable metaphylactic antibiotics on arrival to the feedlot (Personal communication with Dr. Steve Hendrick, Coaldale Vet Clinic, Alberta, Canada). The decision for metaphylactic intervention is primarily based on the nature of cattle population arriving at the feedlot. Cattle populations that are lighter body weight, multiple sources origin, and have poor health history and experienced long distance travel are often subjected to metaphylactic treatment at feedlot entry [26]. Metaphylactic treatment reduces BRD-associated morbidity and mortality by eradicating the already existing bacterial infections and preventing colonization and proliferation of pathogens in those immunosuppressed and vulnerable animals. Although efficacy of metaphylaxis to reduce BRD incidence in feedlots and subsequently improve cattle performance and carcass characteristics has been relatively well documented [26, 27], metaphylaxis is facing more and more public scrutiny due to the increased antimicrobial resistance in BRD pathogens, as well as increased public and scientific concerns regarding the overuse of antimicrobials in livestock production.

Bacterial vaccination is another common practice for the prevention of BRD in feedlot cattle in North America. There are a number of commercial vaccines available against *M. haemolytica*, *P. multocida*, *H. somni* and *M. bovis* [28]. These vaccines are made from bacterins or killed whole bacterium. Bacterial vaccines are less frequently used in feedlots compared to virus vaccines. This might be due to the controversial and limited efficacy of these vaccines against BRD bacterial pathogens [28].

2.3 Current challenges associated with BRD prevention: antimicrobial resistance

Despite advances in antimicrobials and vaccines, increased metaphylactic use and best management efforts to mitigate BRD, the prevalence of BRD in feedlot cattle continues to be increasing [9]. Although data are lacking, one contributor to increased BRD prevalence might be the development and spread of AMR in BRD pathogens. Recent studies have shown the emergence of BRD bacterial pathogens that are resistant to all classes of antibiotics used to treat BRD. For example, *P. multocida* strain isolated from a cow that died of BRD in Alberta has shown resistance up to five different antibiotics commonly used to control BRD (Alexander lab, unpublished data). *M. haemolytica* isolates isolated from Canadian and the US feedlots also exhibited resistance to more than three antibiotics [12, 13, 29]. Multidrug-resistant *H. somni* isolates have also been detected in Albertan feedlots [13].

The prevalence of multidrug-resistant BRD bacterial pathogens is relatively high and increasing in both Canadian and the US feedlots over the years [30]. A recent study conducted in commercial feedlots in Alberta, Canada, revealed that there were significantly high levels of resistance (>70%) against tulathromycin and oxytetracycline in *M. haemolytica* and *P. multocida* isolates and high levels of resistance against oxytetracycline (67%) and penicillin (52%) in *H. somni* isolates isolated from the lower respiratory tract of feedlot cattle with (n = 210) and without (n = 107) BRD [13]. Likewise, Anholt et al. [31] observed that 100% of the *M. haemolytica* (n = 233), *P. multocida* (n = 117) and *M. bovis* (n = 226) and 67% of the *H. somni* (n = 75) isolates isolated from both living and dead BRD-affected cattle, originated from 60 different commercial feedlots in southern Alberta, exhibited resistance towards at least one antimicrobial class. Over 90% of all isolates (n = 745) displayed resistance to macrolide antimicrobials, which are the class of antibiotics commonly used as metaphylaxis. Furthermore, Snyder et al. [14] also reported that a significant increase (from 3.7 to 99.2%) in the prevalence of *M. haemolytica* isolates resistant to tulathromycin in newly received feedlot cattle (n = 169) within 2 weeks after tulathromycin was given as metaphylaxis.

Three or more resistant genes have been detected from *M. haemolytica* and *P. multocida* [15, 29]. These resistant genes are most likely occurring from *de novo* mutation or being acquired from other bacteria. It has been reported that some resistant genes present in BRD bacterial pathogens are being encoded in self-transmissible conjugative elements [15]. Klima et al. [29] identified *M. haemolytica, P. multocida* and *H. somni* isolates from the US and Albertan feedlots that contain integrative conjugative elements (ICE) that conferred resistance up to seven different antimicrobial classes. These ICE can be transferred not only from one BRD pathogens to another BRD pathogen but also to other non-BRD-related bacteria (e.g. *E. coli*) via conjugation [29].

The resistant BRD-related pathogens can not only cause substantial profitability losses to the beef industry and animal welfare issues due to the higher disease relapse and mortality rate but also pose potential threat to the public health given the possibility of these transferable elements carrying resistant genes transfer into zoonotic pathogens. Therefore, counteracting measurements to reduce the development and spread of AMR in BRD pathogens are urgently needed.

3. Alternative antimicrobial approaches to mitigate BRD bacterial pathogens

3.1 Probiotics

Probiotics are defined as "live microorganisms administered in adequate amounts that confer a beneficial health effect on the host" [32]. The scientific recognition of the health-promoting properties of live microbes began in the early 1900s when a Ukrainian scientist, Elias Metchnikoff, hypothesized that the beneficial microbes present in fermented milk could normalize bowel health and prolong life by inhibiting 'putrefactive' bacteria in the gut [32]. Then, lactic acid bacteria (LAB) strains isolated from fermented milk were commercialized with the intention to treat diarrhea in French children in 1906. The term probiotics has been used since 1962. In the past 2 decades, a significant research attention has been given to probiotics, and beneficial effects of probiotics for the mitigation of infections of oral cavity; respiratory, urogenital and gastrointestinal tract [33]; cancer [34] and obesity [35] have been identified.

Bacteria being used as probiotics today include LAB, non-pathogenic *Escherichia coli* and *Bacilli* [36]. The *Lactobacilli* and *Bifidobacteria* genera are the most commonly used as probiotics due to their specific health benefits, high safety profile, and stability [37, 38]. Probiotic bacterium possess unique genetic tools, special membrane structure and composition that allow them to survive under different environmental conditions after ingestion, adhere to the target niche, adapt to special nutrition conditions and integrate with the local microbiota [37].

3.1.1 Mechanisms of probiotic action

Probiotics deliver their beneficial effects to the host through direct inhibition against potential pathogenic bacteria, improving the epithelial barrier function, stimulating the host immune system and re-establishing the commensal microbial community [37]. Probiotic bacteria can directly inhibit pathogens by producing antimicrobial compounds such as lactic acid and bacteriocins. They can also prevent adherence of pathogenic bacteria to the host cells via competitive exclusion, as probiotic strains use the same binding sites as the pathogenic bacteria or downregulate the expression of pathogen-binding sites [37]. Probiotic *Lactobacilli* have also been reported to preserve intestinal epithelial barrier function through stimulating mucin secretion, strengthening tight junction and preventing epithelial cell death and thereby inhibit pathogen translocation [37].

In addition, probiotics have the potential to boost host immune defenses against pathogens by modulating immune response [39]. Probiotics regulate innate and adaptive immune response by modulating immune cells and cytokine production via toll-like receptor-regulated signaling pathways [40]. Probiotic-induced alterations in the functions of dendritic cells, macrophages and T lymphocytes have been documented. For example, probiotic *Lactobacillus* strains modulated dendritic cells and thereby altered cell surface antigen expression and cytokine production in dendritic cells [37, 40]. Additionally, the impact of lactobacillus strains on macrophage function and its TNF-α production capacity has also been reported [41]. Probiotic bacteria *L. acidophilus* influenced the activity of regulatory T cells (Tregs) *in vitro* and *in vivo* in mice [42]. Tregs play a vital role in suppressing inflammation and maintaining immune tolerance.

Modulating the balance of pro- and anti-inflammatory cytokine production is one of the most important mechanisms through which probiotics protect the host from pathogen-induced injury and inflammation [43]. Probiotic bacteria have induced anti-inflammatory cytokine, IL-10, in dendritic and regulatory T cells [43]. IL-10, also known as the master regulator of immunity to infection, plays an essential role in facilitating the optimal pathogen clearance by inhibiting the activity of Th1 cells, NK cells and macrophages [44]. In addition, probiotics inhibit pro-inflammatory cytokine production and thereby prevent excessive inflammation. Probiotic strain *L. rhamnosus* GG inhibited the LPS-stimulated TNF-α production in murine macrophages [45]. Also, *L. rhamnosus* GR-1 strain has significantly or partially reduced LPS-induced number of proinflammatory cytokines including TNF, IFN-γ, IL-1β, IL-2 and IL-6 in human decidual cells [46]. Of note, the immune modulation properties of probiotics are species- and strain-specific, and therefore, different species or different strains within a species are expected to have different immunomodulation properties [37].

The role of probiotics on the local microbiota starts to be better understood due to the completion of the human genome project and the development of next generation DNA sequencing platforms that enabled a deeper understanding of the structure and composition of the host microbiome. Studies suggest that probiotics may re-establish the composition of the gut microbiota and confer beneficial effects on the gut microbial communities [47, 48]. However, there is limited information available with respect to the effects of probiotics on respiratory microbiota. A very recently published study showed that the oral probiotics alter respiratory microbiota of healthy cats [49]. The orally ingested probiotics were detected in the respiratory tract of the cat and were also associated with changes in richness and the overall composition of colonizing microbial populations of the respiratory tract. This observation points out that oral probiotics could alter the respiratory microbiota.

3.1.2 Using probiotics to mitigate BRD bacterial pathogens

Beneficial effects of probiotics in the prevention and control of human respiratory tract infections have been studied. For example, probiotic strain *Streptococcus salivarius* K12 can mitigate pharyngitis by inhibiting the colonization of pathogen

Streptococcus pyogenes and stimulating anti-inflammatory response in epithelial cells [50, 51]. A recent study revealed that the relative abundance of nasopharyngeal LAB in cattle entering the feedlot was significantly greater in animals that remained healthy compared with those that developed BRD [52], suggesting that a certain LAB are important to bovine respiratory mucosal health. Furthermore, an *in vitro* pilot study that we conducted to test antimicrobial properties of commercially available LAB strains (*Lactobacillus*) against *M. haemolytica* demonstrated the possibility of using probiotics to mitigate BRD pathogens [53]. The *Lactobacillus* strains isolated from the nasopharynx of healthy feedlot cattle displayed antimicrobial activity against the growth of *M. haemolytica in vitro* [54]. We also recently reported that the intranasal inoculation of *Lactobacillus* spp. strains inhibits the colonization of *M. haemolytica* S1 into the nasopharynx of dairy calves challenged with *M. haemolytica* S1 (Amat et al., unpublished data). These studies suggest the potential application of probiotics to mitigate BRD bacterial pathogens in feedlot cattle as an alternative to antimicrobial metaphylaxis.

3.2 Essential oils

Essential oils (EOs) from aromatic and medicinal plants are receiving increased scientific attention because of their long history of being sources of natural antimicrobial substances for the treatment of infectious diseases [55]. Thanks to their natural mixture of very complex chemical composition, EOs have shown a broad range of antimicrobial activities against both Gram-negative and Gram-positive bacterial pathogens and have long been used for respiratory tract infections (**Figure 2**) [56, 57]. For example, respiratory pathogens including *Streptococcus pyogenes*, *S. pneumonia* and *Escherichia coli* were effectively inhibited by EOs of cinnamon bark, thyme and spotted beebalm *in vitro* [58].

Interestingly, EOs exhibit minimal effects on LAB including *Lactobacilli* and *Bifidobacteria* that are commonly used as probiotics [59], suggesting EOs may have limited negative effects on beneficial bacteria within the host microbiota. The EOs showed higher minimal inhibition concentration (MIC) values for the probiotic bacteria, whereas it was effective in much lesser concentration against pathogenic bacteria in gastrointestinal tract [59]. Saguibo et al. [60] reported that some probiotic LAB have selective resistance against inhibitory effect of several plant extracts that displayed a strong inhibition on pathogenic bacteria. These evidences suggest the possible combination of the probiotics with EOs and combat with pathogenic bacteria. Probiotics accomplish their antimicrobial activities mainly through producing bacteriocin. In most cases, the probiotics inhibit proliferation of pathogens by generating acidic environment and thereby lower the chance of pathogens' survival. EOs exhibit their antibacterial effect by inducing morphological changes in the target bacterial cells as well as producing reactive oxygen species (ROS) within the bacterial culture [58]. The EOs can accomplish a complete killing of the pathogens even at a lower dosage as the pathogens are normally lack of counteracting mechanism against the effects of EOs [59]. Combining EOs with probiotics is expected to increase the efficacy of probiotics in controlling the bacterial pathogens owing to their synergistic effect which is normally higher than the two individual effects due to their complementary actions [61].

Immune stimulatory effects of EOs have also been well documented. EOs extracted from *Eucalyptus globules* stimulated the innate cell-mediated immune response [62]. Inhibition of cytokine production and arachidonic acid metabolism by a compound of eucalyptus EO has been observed in human blood monocytes *in vitro* [63]. The same authors also reported the anti-inflammatory effects of eucalyptus EO in bronchial asthma [64]. Likewise, vapors of EOs showed

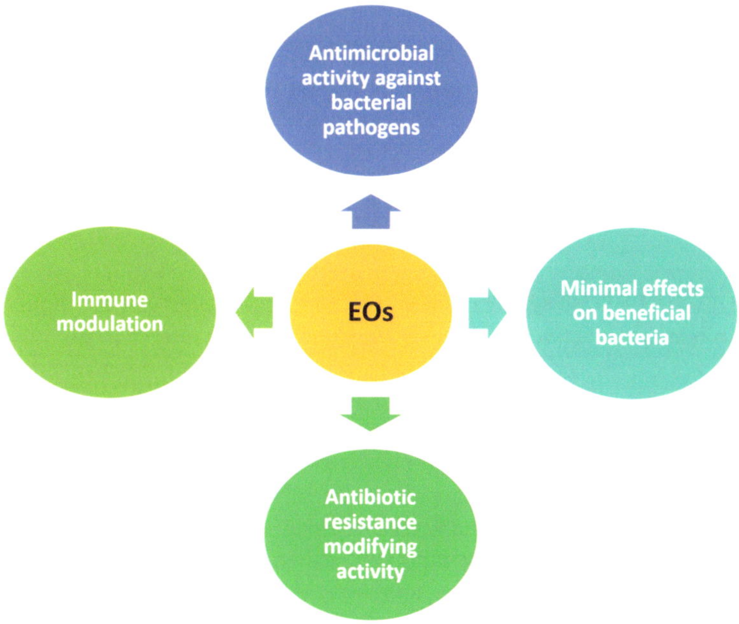

Figure 2.
The antibacterial properties of essential oils (EOs).

anti-inflammatory effect on the trachea and reduced asthma [65]. In addition to the antimicrobial and immune modulation properties, the antibiotic resistance modifying activity of EOs has recently been gaining research interest [66–68]. Some EOs and their major components, such as thymol and geraniol, have shown to improve the efficacy of antibiotics against multidrug-resistant bacterial pathogens and therefore have been suggested to be used as antibiotic adjuvants [67, 69, 70].

3.2.1 Using EOs to mitigate BRD bacterial pathogens

Although antimicrobial activity of EOs against human respiratory bacterial pathogens has been well documented, limited information is available with respect to the effects of EOs against bovine respiratory pathogens. We have recently published data showing that EOs inhibit the BRD bacterial pathogens *M. haemolytica*, *P. multocida* and *H. somni* [16]. The EOs of ajowan, thyme and cinnamon leaf completely or partially inhibited these BRD pathogens in both vapor and liquid phases [16, 17]. These EOs did not display any noticeable cytotoxicity to bovine turbinate cells of the upper respiratory tract [17] and also exhibited minimal antimicrobial activity on six commensal *Lactobacillus* strains that were isolated from the nasal pharynx of a healthy feedlot cattle [17]. This suggests that EOs will have limited negative effects on the commensal bacterial community within the bovine respiratory tract, when they are administered to target pathogens. In addition, Kissels et al. [71] evaluated four different EO components, including carvacrol, thymol, transanethole and 1,8-cineole, as antibacterial agents or as adjuvants for the antibiotics doxycycline and tilmicosin against *M. haemolytica* and *P. multocida*. Carvacrol and thymol inhibited the growth of both of these tested pathogens with MIC values ranged from 0.63 to 2.50 mM. These two EO compounds also displayed an additive effect when one of them was combined with tilmicosin. In addition, combination of thymol with dexycycline displayed synergetic effect against tested BRD pathogens. These studies demonstrated that EOs can be used to control bovine respiratory pathogens in feedlot cattle. Volatile nature of EO makes the EO more promising therapy for the control of bovine respiratory pathogen in the upper respiratory tract as it makes suitable to intranasal administration via nasal spray [72]. However, further research in terms of the effect of EOs on the respiratory commensal microbiota of cattle and the cytotoxicity of EOs on lower respiratory tract is needed.

4. Conclusions

The economic impacts of cattle disease on the beef cattle industry still remain significant, with BRD being the most significant health problem in modern feedlot industry in North America. The BRD is commonly associated with pneumonia in nursing beef calves and recently weaned feedlot cattle and often occurs within the first 45 days after feedlot placement. The BRD is considered as one of the most significant health problems in the beef industry accounting for economic losses that surpass those incurred by all other diseases of cattle combined. Treatment and control of BRD in the beef sector are aimed mainly at bacterial pathogens through antimicrobial use (therapeutic and non-therapeutic administration) and vaccination programs. However, recent studies have shown the emergence of bacterial pathogens associated with BRD that are resistant to all classes of antibiotics used to treat BRD. The increase in the multidrug resistance towards these antimicrobials that are being used as metaphylaxis in feedlots necessitates the development of novel methods to mitigate bovine respiratory pathogens in feedlot cattle as alternatives to metaphylactic antimicrobial use. Probiotic and EOs, being two major natural antimicrobial sources, display the potential application of antimicrobial alternative agents against bovine respiratory bacterial pathogens. More research is needed to develop nasal-delivered probiotics or EOs that can inhibit pathogenic bacteria, with limited effects on commensals and respiratory tract, after intranasal administration.

Acknowledgements

The author thanks his PhD supervisors, Drs. Trevor Alexander and Edouard Timsit, for their supervision. Some of the research work relating to the probiotic and essential oil approaches to mitigate bovine respiratory pathogens discussed in the present chapter is part of the author's PhD project which is funded by the Alberta Livestock and Meat Agency (ALMA). The author also thanks Natural Science and Research Council of Canada for providing a doctoral scholarship. The author also acknowledges Bio-figure for preparing **Figure 1**.

Conflict of interest

No conflict of interest.

Author details

Samat Amat[1,2]*

1 Agriculture and Agri-Food Canada, Lethbridge, AB, Canada

2 Department of Production Animal Health, Faculty of Veterinary Medicine, University of Calgary, Calgary, AB, Canada

*Address all correspondence to: amaiti.saimaiti@agr.gc.ca

IntechOpen

© 2019 The Author(s). Licensee IntechOpen. This chapter is distributed under the terms of the Creative Commons Attribution License (http://creativecommons.org/licenses/by/3.0), which permits unrestricted use, distribution, and reproduction in any medium, provided the original work is properly cited.

References

[1] USDA-NASS. Overview of the United States Cattle Industry (June 2016). SW, Washington, DC: National Agricultural Statistics Service (NASS), Agricultural Statistics Board, United States Department of Agriculture (USDA); 2016

[2] Canada's Beef Industry Fast Facts. https://canadabeef.ca/canadian-beef-industry-fast-facts/; 2016

[3] World Population Statistics. Available from: http://www.worldometers.info/world-population/ [Accessed: 10-10-2017]

[4] Loneragan GH, Thomson DU, Montgomery DL, Mason GL, Larson RL. Prevalence, outcome, and health consequences associated with persistent infection with bovine viral diarrhea virus in feedlot cattle. Journal of the American Veterinary Medical Association. 2005;**226**:595-601

[5] Buhman MJ, Perino LJ, Galyean ML, Wittum TE, Montgomery TH, Swingle RS. Association between changes in eating and drinking behaviors and respiratory tract disease in newly arrived calves at a feedlot. American Journal of Veterinary Research. 2000;**61**:1163-1168

[6] Dargatz D, Lombard J. Summary of BRD data from the 2011 NAHMS feedlot and dairy heifer studies. Animal Health Research Reviews. 2014;**15**(2):123-125. DOI: 10.1017/S1466252314000127

[7] Griffin D. Economic impact associated with respiratory disease in beef cattle. The Veterinary Clinics of North America. Food Animal Practice. 1997;**13**:367-377

[8] Duff GC, Galyean ML. Board-invited review: Recent advances in management of highly stressed, newly received feedlot cattle. Journal of Animal Science. 2007;**85**:823-840

[9] Hilton WM. BRD in 2014: Where have we been, where are we now, and where do we want to go? Animal Health Research Reviews. 2014;**15**:120-122

[10] Griffin D, Chengappa M, Kuszak J, McVey DS. Bacterial pathogens of the bovine respiratory disease complex. The Veterinary Clinics of North America. Food Animal Practice. 2010;**26**:381-394

[11] Edwards TA. Control methods for bovine respiratory disease for feedlot cattle. The Veterinary Clinics of North America. Food Animal Practice. 2010;**26**:273-284

[12] Noyes NR, Benedict KM, Gow SP, et al. *Mannheimia haemolytica* in feedlot cattle: Prevalence of recovery and associations with antimicrobial use, resistance, and health outcomes. Journal of Veterinary Internal Medicine. 2015;**29**:705-713

[13] Timsit E, Hallewell J, Booker C, Tison N, Amat S, Alexander TW. Prevalence and antimicrobial susceptibility of *Mannheimia haemolytica*, *Pasteurella multocida*, and *Histophilus somni* isolated from the lower respiratory tract of healthy feedlot cattle and those diagnosed with bovine respiratory disease. Veterinary Microbiology. 2017;**208**:118-125

[14] Snyder E, Credille B, Berghaus R, Giguere S. Prevalence of multi drug antimicrobial resistance in isolated from high-risk stocker cattle at arrival and two weeks after processing. Journal of Animal Science. 2017;**95**:1124-1131

[15] Portis E, Lindeman C, Johansen L, Stoltman G. A ten-year (2000-2009) study of antimicrobial susceptibility of bacteria that cause bovine respiratory disease complex–*Mannheimia*

haemolytica, *Pasteurella multocida*, and *Histophilus somni*-in the United States and Canada. Journal of Veterinary Diagnostic Investigation. 2012;**24**:932-944

[16] Amat S, Baines D, Alexander TW. A vapor-phase assay for evaluating the antimicrobial activities of essential oils against bovine respiratory bacterial pathogens. Letters in Applied Microbiology. 2017;**65**:489-495. DOI: 10.1111/lam.12804

[17] Amat S, Baines D, Alexander TW. Antimicrobial activities of commercial essential oils against the bovine respiratory pathogen and analysis of their chemical composition and cytotoxicity on bovine turbinate cells (Abstract). Journal of Animal Science. 2017;**95**(supplement 4):122

[18] Taylor JD, Fulton RW, Lehenbauer TW, Step DL, Confer AW. The epidemiology of bovine respiratory disease: What is the evidence for preventive measures? The Canadian Veterinary Journal. 2010;**51**(12):1351-1359

[19] Townsend HG, Meek AH, Lesnick TG, Janzen ED. Factors associated with average daily gain, fever and lameness in beef bulls at the Saskatchewan Central Feed Test Station. Canadian Journal of Veterinary Research. 1989;**53**:349-354

[20] Sanderson MW, Dargatz DA, Wagner BA. Risk factors for initial respiratory disease in United States' feedlots based on producer-collected daily morbidity counts. The Canadian Veterinary Journal. 2008;**49**:373-378

[21] Grissett GP, White BJ, Larson RL. Structured literature review of responses of cattle to viral and bacterial pathogens causing bovine respiratory disease complex. Journal of Veterinary Internal Medicine. 2015;**29**:770-780

[22] Korten I, Mika M, Klenja S, et al. Interactions of respiratory viruses and the nasal microbiota during the first year of life in healthy infants. mSphere. 2016;**1**(6):e00312-e00316. DOI: 10.1128/mSphere.00312-16

[23] Rice JA, Carrasco-Medina L, Hodgins DC, Shewen PE. *Mannheimia haemolytica* and bovine respiratory disease. Animal Health Research Reviews. 2007;**8**:117-128

[24] Klima CL, Alexander TW, Hendrick S, McAllister TA. Characterization of *Mannheimia haemolytica* isolated from feedlot cattle that were healthy or treated for bovine respiratory disease. Canadian Journal of Veterinary Research. 2014;**78**(1):38-45

[25] Klima CL, Cook SR, Zaheer R, et al. Comparative genomic analysis of *Mannheimia haemolytica* from bovine sources. PLoS One. 2016;**11**:e0149520. DOI: 10.1371/journal.pone.0149520

[26] Ives SE, Richeson JT. Use of antimicrobial metaphylaxis for the control of bovine respiratory disease in high-risk cattle. The Veterinary Clinics of North America. Food Animal Practice. 2015;**31**:341-350

[27] Nickell JS, White BJ. Metaphylactic antimicrobial therapy for bovine respiratory disease in stocker and feedlot cattle. The Veterinary Clinics of North America. Food Animal Practice. 2010;**26**:285-301

[28] Larson RL, Step DL. Evidence-based effectiveness of vaccination against *mannheimia haemolytica*, *pasteurella multocida*, and *histophilus somni* in feedlot cattle for mitigating the incidence and effect of bovine respiratory disease complex. The Veterinary Clinics of North America. Food Animal Practice. 2012;**28**:97-106

[29] Klima CL, Zaheer R, Cook SR, et al. Pathogens of bovine respiratory disease

in North American feedlots conferring multidrug resistance via integrative conjugative elements. Journal of Clinical Microbiology. 2014;**52**(2):438-448

[30] Cameron A, McAllister TA. Antimicrobial usage and resistance in beef production. Journal of Animal Science and Biotechnology. 2016;**7**:68-016-0127-3

[31] Anholt RM, Klima C, Allan N, et al. Antimicrobial susceptibility of bacteria that cause bovine respiratory disease complex in Alberta, Canada. Frontiers in Veterinary Science. 2017;**4**:207. DOI: 10.3389/fvets.2017.00207

[32] Joint FAO/WHO Working Group Report on Drafting Guidelines for the Evaluation of Probiotics in Food London, Ontario, Canada. April 30 and May 1, 2002

[33] Caramia G, Silvi S. Probiotics: From the ancient wisdom to the actual therapeutical perspective. In: Malago JJ, Koninkx JFJG, Marinsek-Logar R, editors. Probiotic Bacteria and Enteric Infections. Dordrecht: Springer; 2011. pp. 3-38. ISBN 978-94-007-0385-8

[34] Yu AQ Li L. The potential role of probiotics in cancer prevention and treatment. Nutrition and Cancer. 2016;**68**:535-544

[35] Kobyliak N, Conte C, Cammarota G, et al. Probiotics in prevention and treatment of obesity: A critical view. Nutrition & Metabolism (London). 2016;**13**:14-016-0067-0. eCollection 2016

[36] Fijan S. Microorganisms with claimed probiotic properties: An overview of recent literature. International Journal of Environmental Research and Public Health. 2014;**11**(5):4745-4767

[37] Lebeer S, Vanderleyden J, De Keersmaecker SCJ. Genes and molecules of Lactobacilli supporting probiotic action. Microbiology and Molecular Biology Reviews. 2008;**72**(4):728-764

[38] Bogovič-Matijašić B, Rogelj I. Bacteriocins of probiotics and enteric cytoprotection. In: Malago JJ, Koninkx JFJG, Marinsek-Logar R, editors. Probiotic Bacteria and Enteric Infections. Dordrecht: Springer; 2011. pp. 313-354. ISBN 978-94-007-0385-8

[39] Kemgang TS, Kapila S, Shanmugam VP, Kapila R. Cross-talk between probiotic lactobacilli and host immune system. Journal of Applied Microbiology. 2014;**117**:303-319

[40] Malago JJ, Koninkx JFJG. Modulation of immune system by probiotics to protect against enteric disorders. In: Malago JJ, Koninkx JFJG, Marinsek-Logar R, editors. Probiotic Bacteria and Enteric Infections. Dordrecht: Springer; 2011. pp. 263-286. ISBN 978-94-007-0385-8

[41] Kim SO, Sheikh HI, Ha SD, Martins A, Reid G. G-CSF-mediated inhibition of JNK is a key mechanism for *Lactobacillus rhamnosus*-induced suppression of TNF production in macrophages. Cellular Microbiology. 2006;**8**:1958-1971

[42] Petersen ER, Claesson MH, Schmidt EG, et al. Consumption of probiotics increases the effect of regulatory T cells in transfer colitis. Inflammatory Bowel Diseases. 2012;**18**:131-142

[43] Vanderpool C, Yan F, Polk DB. Mechanisms of probiotic action: Implications for therapeutic applications in inflammatory bowel diseases. Inflammatory Bowel Diseases. 2008;**14**:1585-1596

[44] Couper KN, Blount DG, Riley EM. IL-10: The master regulator of immunity to infection. Journal of Immunology. 2008;**180**:5771-5777

[45] Pena JA, Versalovic J. *Lactobacillus rhamnosus* GG decreases TNF-alpha production in lipopolysaccharide-activated murine macrophages by a contact-independent mechanism. Cellular Microbiology. 2003;**5**:277-285

[46] Li W, Yang S, Kim SO, Reid G, Challis JR, Bocking AD. Lipopolysaccharide-induced profiles of cytokine, chemokine, and growth factors produced by human decidual cells are altered by lactobacillus rhamnosus GR-1 supernatant. Reproductive Sciences. 2014;**21**:939-947

[47] Hemarajata P, Versalovic J. Effects of probiotics on gut microbiota: Mechanisms of intestinal immunomodulation and neuromodulation. Therapeutic Advances in Gastroenterology. 2013;**6**:39-51

[48] Sanchez B, Delgado S, Blanco-Miguez A, Lourenco A, Gueimonde M, Margolles A. Probiotics, gut microbiota, and their influence on host health and disease. Molecular Nutrition & Food Research. 2017;**61**. DOI: 10.1002/mnfr.201600240. Epub 2016 Oct 10

[49] Vientos-Plotts AI, Ericsson AC, Rindt H, Reinero CR. Oral probiotics alter healthy feline respiratory microbiota. Frontiers in Microbiology. 2017;**8**:1287

[50] Kreikemeyer B, McIver KS, Podbielski A. Virulence factor regulation and regulatory networks in *Streptococcus pyogenes* and their impact on pathogen-host interactions. Trends in Microbiology. 2003;**11**:224-232. DOI: 10.1016/S0966-842X(03)00098-2

[51] Cosseau C, Devine DA, Dullaghan E, et al. The commensal *Streptococcus salivarius* K12 downregulates the innate immune responses of human epithelial cells and promotes host-microbe homeostasis. Infection and Immunity. 2008;**76**:4163-4175

[52] Holman DB, McAllister TA, Topp E, Wright AD, Alexander TW. The nasopharyngeal microbiota of feedlot cattle that develop bovine respiratory disease. Veterinary Microbiology. 2015;**180**:90-95

[53] Amat S, Subramanian S, Timsit E, Alexander TW. Probiotic bacteria inhibit the bovine respiratory pathogen *Mannheimia haemolytica* serotype 1 in vitro. Letters in Applied Microbiology. 2017;**64**:343-349

[54] Amat S, Timsit E, Holman DB, Alexander TW. 0472 characterization of bovine nasopharyngeal lactic acid bacteria and their in vitro antimicrobial activities against the respiratory pathogen *Mannheimia haemolytica*. Journal of Animal Science. 2016;**96**(suppl_5):225-226

[55] Nabavi SM, Marchese A, Izadi M, Curti V, Daglia M, Nabavi SF. Plants belonging to the genus Thymus as antibacterial agents: From farm to pharmacy. Food Chemistry. 2015;**173**:339-347

[56] Fabio A, Cermelli C, Fabio G, Nicoletti P, Quaglio P. Screening of the antibacterial effects of a variety of essential oils on microorganisms responsible for respiratory infections. Phytotherapy Research. 2007;**21**:374-377

[57] Cermelli C, Fabio A, Fabio G, Quaglio P. Effect of eucalyptus essential oil on respiratory bacteria and viruses. Current Microbiology. 2008;**56**:89-92

[58] Li H, Yang T, Li FY, Yao Y, Sun ZM. Antibacterial activity and mechanism of action of *Monarda punctata* essential oil and its main components against common bacterial pathogens in respiratory tract. International Journal of Clinical and Experimental Pathology. 2014;**7**:7389-7398

[59] Hawrelak JA, Cattley T, Myers SP. Essential oils in the treatment of intestinal dysbiosis: A preliminary in vitro study. Alternative Medicine Review. 2009;**14**:380-384

[60] Saguibo JD, Elegado FB. Resistance profile of probiotic lactic acid bacteria against inhibitory effects of selected plant extracts. The Philippine Agricultural Scientist. 2012;**95**:22-32

[61] Shipradeep SK, Khare RS, Ojha S, Kundu K, Kundu S. Development of probiotic candidate in combination with essential oils from medicinal plant and their effect on enteric pathogens: A review. Gastroenterology Research and Practice. 2012;**2012**:457150

[62] Serafino A, Vallebona PS, Andreola F, et al. Stimulatory effect of Eucalyptus essential oil on innate cell-mediated immune response. BMC Immunology. 2008;**9**:17. DOI: 10.1186/1471-2172-9-17

[63] Juergens UR, Stober M, Vetter H. Inhibition of cytokine production and arachidonic acid metabolism by eucalyptol (1,8-cineole) in human blood monocytes in vitro. European Journal of Medical Research. 1998;**3**:508-510

[64] Juergens UR, Dethlefsen U, Steinkamp G, Gillissen A, Repges R, Vetter H. Anti-inflammatory activity of 1.8-cineol (eucalyptol) in bronchial asthma: A double-blind placebo-controlled trial. Respiratory Medicine. 2003;**97**:250-256

[65] Frohlich H. Long–range coherence and energy storage in biological system. International Journal of Quantum Chemistry. 1968;**2**:641-649

[66] Fankam AG, Kuiate JR, Kuete V. Antibacterial and antibiotic resistance modifying activity of the extracts from *Allanblackia gabonensis*, *Combretum molle* and *Gladiolus quartinianus* against gram-negative bacteria including multi-drug resistant phenotypes. BMC Complementary and Alternative Medicine. 2015;**15**:206-015-0726-0

[67] Yap PS, Krishnan T, Yiap BC, Hu CP, Chan KG, Lim SH. Membrane disruption and anti-quorum sensing effects of synergistic interaction between *Lavandula angustifolia* (lavender oil) in combination with antibiotic against plasmid-conferred multi-drug-resistant *Escherichia coli*. Journal of Applied Microbiology. 2014;**116**:1119-1128

[68] Yap PS, Yiap BC, Ping HC, Lim SH. Essential oils, a new horizon in combating bacterial antibiotic resistance. The Open Microbiology Journal. 2014;**8**:6-14

[69] Lorenzi V, Muselli A, Bernardini AF, Berti L, Pages JM, Amaral L, et al. Geraniol restores antibiotic activities against multidrug-resistant isolates from gram-negative species. Antimicrobial Agents and Chemotherapy. 2009;**53**:2209-2211

[70] Veras HNH, Rodrigues FFG, Botelho MA, Menezes IRA, Coutinho HDM, Costa JGM. Enhancement of aminoglycosides and β-lactams antibiotic activity by essential oil of Lippia sidoides Cham. and the Thymol. Arabian Journal of Chemistry. 2017;**10**:S2790-S2795

[71] Kissels W, Wu X, Santos RR. Short communication: Interaction of the isomers carvacrol and thymol with the antibiotics doxycycline and tilmicosin: In vitro effects against pathogenic bacteria commonly found in the respiratory tract of calves. Journal of Dairy Science. 2017;**100**(2):970-974

[72] Inouye S, Takizawa T, Yamaguchi H. Antibacterial activity of essential oils and their major constituents against respiratory tract pathogens by gaseous contact. The Journal of Antimicrobial Chemotherapy. 2001;**47**:565-573

Section 3

Major Bacterial Causes of Abortion in Cows

Chapter 3

One Health Approach to Control Brucellosis in Sierra Leone

Roland Suluku, Jesse P.J. Nyandeboh and Sheku Moiforay

Abstract

Brucellosis is a febrile zoonotic disease that presents a severe hazard to humans and domestic animals, which requires a One Health approach to control socioeconomic consequences and public health implications on the people in the country. The majority of the cattle owners are illiterate herds' men with traditional knowledge of cattle management handed down by their ancestors. Management is free range with no supplementing or balanced diet. Access to veterinary services is almost not available, and local herdsmen treat their animals. Most of these herdsmen do not allow livestock officer visitors to have access to their animals. Processing of meat and milk uses traditional methods, and people consume fresh milk without due regard to sanitary conditions. This behavior has serious public health implications especially when the majority of the beneficiaries live in rural communities. Animals abort, while production decreases due to delayed conception. Local herdsmen confer confidence in people who are knowledgeable about cattle management. Researchers have no data on the disease in the last 50 years. Supportive action from various sectors such as human, animal and environmental health stakeholders backed by social anthropologists using the One Health Platform will provide a conducive atmosphere to engage herdsmen in initiating control measures of the disease.

Keywords: brucellosis, herdsmen, animals, community, One Health

1. Introduction

Brucellosis is a common contagious, communicable and One Health endemic zoonotic disease of public health significance with a high rate of morbidity and life sterility [1]. Brucellosis is named after Sir David Bruce because he isolated the causative agent from a soldier while working in Malta. The disease Malta *fever* or *Mediterranean fever* got it named when it affected British military personnel in 1886. Malta fever is a fever condition occasionally caused by *Brucella*, and its most common species *B. abortus* and *B. melitensis*. *B. abortus* causes premature delivery in cattle and intermittent fever in human [2, 3].

1.1 Animals affected

Brucellosis is a bacterial disease of the genus *Brucella*, and six different species exist; namely:

i. *B. abortus*

ii. *B. melitensis*

iii. *B. suis*

iv. *B canis*

v. *B. ovis*

vi. *B. neotomae*—desert rat

The disease affects cattle, goat, sheep, pigs, buffaloes, camels and reindeer, and other animals may be less frequently affected. All the above diseases cause *brucellosis*, but of significance to man and animals worldwide are three species *Brucella suis* affecting pigs, *Brucella melitensis* affecting small ruminants and *Brucella abortus* affecting cattle. *Brucella canis* also affects dogs.

Recent research shows that Brucella causes pinnipedialis in seals and *ceti* sp. in whales [4].

1.2 Socioeconomic effect of brucellosis

Brucella causes abortion in pregnant cow or premature calving, death of young animals, birth of weak calves, stillbirth, delayed calving, sterility, retained placenta, male infertility followed by a decrease in milk yield [1, 5]. The death is due to *mastitis* and *hygromas* in African cattle. *Vesiculitis, epididymis* and *orchitis* are characteristic in the bull which sometimes leads to *testicular abscesses, metritis* and life infertility. In pregnant animals, a visible swelling of the mammary gland around the naval region followed by bleeding from the vagina is not common in pregnant animals infected with *Brucella*. Enlargement of the udder indicates a high level of bacteria in shredded milk, urine and vagina discharge.

1.3 Transmission of bovine brucellosis

1.3.1 Animal

Bacteria are excreted with the fetus, the placenta and uterine fluid during calving.

Animals' discharge the organism after parturition, abortion or via milk of infected cow [6, 7].

Infected breeding bulls transmit infection via semen.

Vertical transmission is through calves or lamb in the uterus [1, 8].

Transmission can occur through contaminated water and feed.

1.3.2 Humans

Human *brucellosis* has different names based on the region in which the disease occurred. They named it *Malta fever*, because Dr. Bruce discovered the disease in this town, *Cyprus or Mediterranean fever*, *rocky fever of Gibraltar*, *intermitted typhoid* and *undulant fever* [9, 10].

Fever is a general symptom across all human patients. Uterus infection with fetal death accompanied by general malaise, fatigue and arthritis with chronic and recurring febrility with joint pain are common in human beings [10, 11]. Chronic symptoms include loss of working day, high fever because of septicemia followed by emancipation, insomnia, headache, loss of appetite and sexual impotence in a human patient [12].

Human to human transmission occurs through transplacenta and breastfeeding but not through sexual intercourse, blood transfusion or transplantation of body organs [10, 13]. The disease is transmitted by direct contact with infected tissue or their products [10, 11]. Transmission by inhalation of an organism or into the conjunctiva occurs by air. In humans, transmission is not limited to the reproductive organs but the nervous system. It causes *neurobrucellosis* showing symptoms of *meningitis*, *encephalitis*, *stroke*, *myelitis* and *neuropsychiatric* features [14]. *Brucellosis* causes deafness as reported by other scientists [15].

1.4 Africa and Asia

Brucellosis is one of the most widespread bacterial zoonotic diseases in the world. It affects both humans and domestic and wild animals [16]. WHO reports about 500,000 cases of human brucellosis every year [17]. An economic impact assessment conducted in both Africa and Asia in 2013 by McDermott et al. [18] shows that the disease is endemic across Africa and Asia continents and responsible for most of the human cases. The disease worsens and deprives people in developing countries like sub-Saharan Africa of the much-needed protein. Poverty is a driving force of brucellosis especially in communities where people depend heavily on livestock for their livelihood [19].

Brucella subtype causes brucellosis in many parts of the world including West Africa. *Brucella abortus biovar* 3 is a common strain that affects cattle [20]. These West African isolates are mostly characterized from autochthonous cattle and hygroma fluid samples. Data are required to assess the potential threats of public health importance both at national and regional levels.

2. Brucellosis in Sierra Leone

Sierra Leone is located in the humid tropical forest in the west coast of West Africa. It is boarded by the Republic of Guinea in the north and north-west and Liberia in the south and southwest and by the Atlantic Ocean in the west. The country has five ecological zones: the Mangrove swamp, Savannah grassland, forest vegetation, inland valley swamp and Bolland and has nine significant rivers that retain water all year round.

The high natural vegetation provides a conducive environment for rearing animals such as ruminants. Ruminant production such as cattle is confined to the northern district of Koinadugu extending north-eastward to Kono District and southward to Bombali District. These three districts were known as the cattle belt of Sierra Leone. Major cattle markets exist in these districts.

Brucellosis outbreak occurred in Sierra Leone in 1966. The veterinary division mounted a campaign, which they divided into three phases, from 1966 to 1969. About 50% of herds became infected in Bombali and Kono, and cases of abortion were reported in Njala. Strain 19 has been used over the years, but the problem persists. A nationwide vaccination and DCIP Havac strain (45/20) were anticipated, but never materialized.

Most of the veterinary structures and institutions started degenerating during this period. The status of the disease remains unknown, but abortion and stillbirth are common among ruminants throughout the country.

Estimated number of livestock by type, district and region						
Administrative units	**Type**					
	Cattle	**Goat**	**Sheep**	**Pigs**	**Chickens**	**Ducks**
District						
Kailahun	430	54,478	17,159	6924	98,894	150
Kenema	5332	73,507	50,980	11,842	200,560	25,861
Kono	101,156	44,661	22,559	5455	65,599	3675
Bombali	158,705	61,723	51,831	8553	125,451	2623
Kambia	62,223	47,053	26,503	6278	171,903	3305
Koinadugu	97,858	63,327	39,136	38,214	137,045	630
Port Loko	11,614	97,596	52,737	4909	259,212	5436
Tonkolili	36,138	76,796	31,744	5047	115,903	2398
Bo	50,930	97,920	22,640	9086	173,037	10,493
Bonthe	6840	26,987	9161	9051	60,715	12,078
Moyamba	11,629	48,101	8499	5660	146,996	7606
Pujehun	3510	36,934	28,136	5265	86,335	8352
WAR&U**	514	83,822	66,581	101,213	314,981	17,167
Total	**546,881**	**812,906**	**427,667**	**217,497**	**1,956,630**	**99,775**
Region						
Eastern	106,918	172,646	90,698	24,221	365,053	29,686
Northern	366,539	346,495	201,951	63,001	809,513	14,392
Southern	72,911	209,942	68,436	29,062	467,082	38,530
Western Area	514	83,822	66,581	101,214	314,981	17,168
Total	**546,881**	**812,906**	**427,667**	**217,497**	**1,956,630**	**99,775**

*Source: [22]. **Western Area Rural & Urban.*

Table 1.
Projections for national livestock populations by species, by district and by region.

Table 1 explains the increase and spread of cattle production from the north and east in 1966 [21] to every district in the country [22]. This spread of cattle production corresponds to an increase in the spread of brucellosis. The majority of cattle owners or herders are Fulani nomads with little or no formal education. Pastoral Fulani who own approximately 90% of the national herd [23] own cattle production.

The majority of the cattle owners practice a free-range animal production system, which encourages animals to move into large areas of land in search of food. Pastoralists utilize an extensive range of land as common pool resources through movement from one location to another making full use of their character and cultural practices [24]. In Nigeria, land use management is characterized by the transhumant system due to vegetation variations, agricultural practices and tsetse fly infestation [25]. Fulani pastoralists migrated to Hausa land from Senegalese valley in western Sudan but were forced to move due to deteriorating environmental conditions, land degradation and recurrent draught, thus accounting for the exodus to Guinea savannah to the forest fringes in the southern parts of Nigeria [26].

Illiteracy is a significant factor among cattle herds or agropastoralists exacerbating brucellosis or other cattle diseases in West Africa and Sierra Leone in particular. Cattle rearers or agropastoralists use knowledge passed onto them by their accentors. Studies conducted in northern Nigeria reported a common feature of rural farming, as about 42% of cattle rearers or agropastoralists are illiterate or had no formal education [27]. The majority of pastoralists (58%) had no western formal education compared to 66.2% who had acquired Islamic education [28]. As a result, they have no balanced diet prepared for their animals, nor supplementation of the ration. Kassam [29] opined that the livestock sector lacks adequate supplies of quality feed and pasture.

Animals became malnourished, emaciated and exposed to diseases. Compounding the situation further is the lack of adequate veterinary service to attend to the needed problems of the cattle herds. One of the main problems highlighted by cattle farmers is the lack of poor veterinary services available in their communities [30]. Cattle farmers purchase drugs from foot peddlers to treat their animals. All the cattle ranches visited in Sierra Leone have drugs to treat their animals. Cattle farmers refuse government officials or livestock officer access to their animals.

Cattle milk is a significant source of brucellosis. When people pasteurize milk, they reduce human infection. Resource-limited or poor communities do not pasteurize milk due to their long-standing traditional beliefs and cultural practices and the complete lack of public health implications of raw milk consumption [31]. These food products from the informal sector escape formal health and safety practices, thereby increasing the spread of brucellosis to the general public [32].

3. How do we control brucellosis in Sierra Leone?

The strategy to prevent brucellosis is much dependent on the production system. Two methods used include test and slaughter and vaccination. The former requires a laboratory facility, which is lacking in the rural communities. The latter option involves not only the administration of vaccines but also many other techniques and includes various sectors of people.

A large percentage of the adult population in Sierra Leone is illiterate and live in rural communities where cattle farmers exist. Any change or transformation in the cattle sector to control brucellosis will require the involvement of the entire cattle rearers and the community people. This approach is known as One Health.

One Health approach is any benefit to the complete well-being of humans, animals and their environment because of the synergy of integrated humans, and veterinary is a positive step toward the One Health approach. Such vale can even include financial savings and environmental services [33].

The One Health approach involves the following:

i. Conducting a scoping mission to ascertain the prevalence and incidence of the disease in the community. It involves visiting communities where the disease has occurred and identifying stakeholders for future discussion on an agreed date based on their farming calendar. It also includes gaining knowledge about the sociocultural and traditional customs of the people in a defined community.

ii. Holding stakeholder meetings with animal rearers and owners including local administrative authorities in the community. In this forum, the scoping team meets the local administration to tell them about the etiology and epidemiology of the disease, its mode of transmission, signs and symptoms and how to prevent and control. The local authorities will put a mechanism in place to ensure compliance by all people. This involves both animals' owners and community people, hence the One Health concept.

iii. Engaging community people to identify control and preventive strategies, and ensuring that they understand the process. At this stage, the scoping team members ask community people about existing strategies they have used in the past and how do they intend to control and prevent subsequent outbreaks. Scoping team members equally provide alternative ways based on their experience to control and prevent the disease. Community people select those among various alternatives that suit their needs the most. Local authorities will now engage their people and animal owners to ensure that they understand the controlled strategy. Defaulters pay minimum fine proposed by all.

iv. Identifying the leading players in the prevention of brucellosis. In any community, some people can mobilize the people. Such people known as critical stakeholders command respect in the community; scoping team work with local authorities to identify such people, charge them with the responsibility of passing the message across the community and encourage people to implement the decision of the community in full.

v. Dividing the group into various units or components. Key stakeholders and scoping team members work together and spread the message in the community on the disease which includes the following:

- Print and electronic media. Identifying people within and outside the community to write about the disease and intervention by the community people. Such interventions could be flyers on various aspects of the disease as an awareness-raising process strategy to inform the people and country as a whole.

- Play/drama committee: Identifying people within and outside the community, to act a play on brucellosis. Such play focuses mainly on how people contract the disease, signs and symptoms, mode of transmission, prevention and control. The drama target public health aspects of eating dead animals with the disease. Such interventions will educate the public and communities will put the disease under control.

- Songs: They composed songs in their local dialect as a means of understanding the disease correctly.

- Quiz committee for schoolchildren. Quiz competitions are held in various schools where the outbreak has occurred; children pass the message to their parents and neighbors from the competitions held. Such actions will educate the general populace and help reduce or eradicate it from the community.

- Bike riders, taxi/poda poda drivers: These are a group or community of people who aid in killing and stealing of these animals in the community. Involving them in the awareness campaign and the implementation of the provisions of the by-laws will reduce stealing and minimize the spread of the disease. In such communities no bike rider transports animals after 6:00 pm.

- Vaccination and registration committee. This committee is charged with the responsibility of educating the people and animal owners about the need to vaccinate their animals. They mount such campaign for about a month or 2 weeks depending on the availability of funds. People bring their animals in large numbers during the vaccination exercise. People register their animals in order to track them during subsequent registration.

- Engaging the radio in massive sensitization and education about brucellosis. The 11 year old civil war made the majority of Sierra Leoneans learn to love to listen to the radio. Such a medium has been used to pass information to the broader public, while at the same time allows them to ask a question. The outbreak of disease has reduced due to increase in knowledge of the people on a particular disease.

vi. Formulating by-laws to ensure compliance by all categories of people and conducting routine vaccination on yearly basis. This bottom-top approach will help in the prevention of brucellosis in Sierra Leone.

vii. The above process benefits people by engaging them all in fighting disease outbreaks. Such gathering of people to fight the common enemy called disease is known as ONE HEALTH.

4. Conclusions

Brucellosis is a zoonotic disease ravaging resource-poor communities in the world including Africa and Asia. Vaccination campaigns in Sierra Leone had not eradicated the disease since 1966. The One Health approach which adds value to people's lives by the involvement of all partners with a strong medium of communication is a step in the right direction toward controlling the disease in Sierra Leone.

Conflict of interest

The authors have not declared any conflict of interest.

Author details

Roland Suluku*, Jesse P.J. Nyandeboh and Sheku Moiforay
Njala University, Njala, Sierra Leone

*Address all correspondence to: nyasulukuroland2710@gmail.com

IntechOpen

© 2019 The Author(s). Licensee IntechOpen. This chapter is distributed under the terms of the Creative Commons Attribution License (http://creativecommons.org/licenses/by/3.0), which permits unrestricted use, distribution, and reproduction in any medium, provided the original work is properly cited.

References

[1] ZKI M, Muhammad Z. An overview of brucellosis in cattle and humans, and its serological and molecular diagnosis in control strategies. Tropical Medicine and Infectious Diseases. 2018;**3**(2):65

[2] Cutler SJ, Whitmore AM, Commander NJ. Brucellosis—New aspects of an old disease. Journal of Applied Microbiology. 2005;**98**:1270-1281

[3] Christopher S, Umapathy B, Ravikumar K. Brucellosis: Review on the recent trends in pathogenicity and laboratory diagnosis. Journal of Laboratory Physicians. 2010;**2**:55-60

[4] Foster G, Osterman SB, Godfroid J, Jacques I, Cloeckaert A. *Brucella ceti* sp. nov. Moreover, *Brucella pinnipedialis* sp. nov. for Brucella strains with cetaceans and seals as their preferred hosts. International Journal of Systematic and Evolutionary Microbiology. 2007;**57**:2688-2693

[5] Garofolo G, Fasanella A, Di Giannatale E, Platone I, Sacchini L, Persiani T, et al. Cases of human brucellosis in Sweden linked to the Middle East and Africa. BMC Research Notes. 2016;**9**:277

[6] Godfroid J, Cloeckaert A, Liautard PJ, Kohler S, Fortin D, Walravens K, et al. From the discovery of the Malta fever's agent to the discovery of a marine mammal reservoir, brucellosis has continuously been a re-emerging zoonosis. Veterinary Research. 2005;**36**:313-326

[7] Ferrero MC, Hielpos SM, Carvalho BN, Barrionuevo P, Corsetti PP, Giambartolomei HG, et al. Key role of toll-like receptor 2 in the inflammatory response and major histocompatibility complex class ii downregulation in *Brucella abortus*-infected alveolar macrophages. Infection and Immunity. 2014;**82**:626-639

[8] Rossetti CA, Arenas-Gamboa AM, Maurizio E. Caprine brucellosis: A historically neglected disease with significant impact on public health. PLoS Neglected Tropical Diseases. 2017;**11**:e0005692

[9] Buzgan T, Karahocagil KM, Irmak H, Baran IA, Karsen H, Evirgen O, et al. Clinical manifestations and complications in 1028 cases of brucellosis: A retrospective evaluation and review of the literature. International Journal of Infectious Diseases. 2010;**14**:e469-e478

[10] Franc KA et al. Brucellosis remains a neglected disease in the developing world: A call for interdisciplinary action. BMC Public HealthBMC series—open, inclusive and trusted. 2018;**18**:125. DOI: 10.1186/s12889-017-5016-y

[11] Kose S, Serin Senger S, Akkoclu G, Kuzucu L, Ulu Y, Ersan G, et al. Clinical manifestations, complications, and treatment of brucellosis: Evaluation of 72 cases. Turkish Journal of Medical Sciences. 2014;**44**(2):220-223. DOI: 10.3906/sag-1112-34

[12] Franco MP, Mulder M, Gilman HR, Smits LH. Human brucellosis. The Lancet Infectious Diseases. 2007;**7**:775-786

[13] Tuon FF, Gondolfo RB, Cerchiari N. Human-to-human transmission of Brucella—A systematic review. Tropical Medicine and International Health. 2017;**22**(5):539-546. DOI: 10.1111/tmi.12856

[14] Gunduz T, Texture TP, Yapici Z, Kurtuncu M, Somer A, Torun MS, et al. Characteristics of isolated spinal cord involvement in neurobrucellosis with no corresponding MRI activity: A case report and review of the literature. Journal of the Neurological Sciences. 2017;**372**:305-306

[15] Ducrotoy MJ, Muñoz MP, Conde-Álvarez R, Blasco MJ, Moriyón I. A systematic review of current immunological tests for the diagnosis of cattle brucellosis. Preventive Veterinary Medicine. 2018;**151**:57-72

[16] Corbel MJ. Brucellosis in Humans and Animals. Geneva: World Health Organization (WHO); 2006

[17] Pappas G, Papadimitriou P, Akritidis N, Christou L, Tsianos EV. The new global map of human brucellosis. The Lancet Infectious Diseases. 2006;**6**:91-99. DOI: 10.1016/S1473-3099(06)70382-6

[18] McDermott J et al. Economics of brucellosis impact and control in low-income countries. Revue Scientifique et Technique. 2013;**32**(1):249-261

[19] Cáceres SB. Comparative veterinary capacity in Western Africa: Implications for livestock development. Livestock Research for Rural Development. 2010. Available from: http://www.lrrd.org/lrrd22/10/burg22180.htm [Accessed: May 26, 2017]

[20] Sanogo M, Abatih E, Thys E, Fretin D, Berkvens D, Saegerman C. Importance of identification and typing of Brucellae from West African cattle: A review. Veterinary Microbiology. 28 Jun 2013;**164**(3-4):202-211. DOI: 10.1016/j.vetmic.2013.02.009. Epub 2013 Feb 26 PMID10.10

[21] Veterinary record 1951. Ministry of Agriculture and Natural Resources

[22] Kwaku A, Mohamed M, Mohamed B. Sierra Leone National Livestock Sample Survey, 2016; 2017

[23] Suleiman H. Policy issues on agropastoral development in Nigeria. In: Proceedings of National Conference on Pastoralism in Nigeria. Zaria, Nigeria: Ahmadu Bello University; 1988

[24] Kaye-Zwiebel E, King E. Kenyan pastoralist societies in transition: Varying perceptions of the value of ecosystem services. Ecology and Society. 2014;**19**(3):17. DOI: 10.5751/ES-06753-190317

[25] Iyayi EA et al. Livestock production pattern of agro-pastoralists in peri-urban centres of south-west Nigeria. Nigerian Journal of Animal Production. 2003;**30**:87-92

[26] Fabusoro E. Critical issues in livelihoods Security of migrant Fulani pastoralist: Empirical evidence from Southwest Nigeria. In: AEGIS European Conference on African studies—African Alternatives: Initiative and creativity beyond current constraints. Leiden, The Netherlands: African Studies Centre; 2007

[27] Adisa RS, Oluwasegun AA. Farmer-herdsmen conflicts: A factor analysis of socio-economic conflict variables among arable crop farmers in North Central Nigeria. Journal of Human Ecology (Delhi, India). 2010;**30**(1):1-9. DOI: 10.1080/09709274.2010.11906266

[28] Dimelu MU, Salifu DE, Enwelu AI, Igbokwe EM. Challenges of herdsmen-farmers' conflict in livestock production in Nigeria: Experience of pastoralists in Kogi State, Nigeria. African Journal of Agricultural Research. 2017;**12**(8):642-650

[29] Kassam A, Kueneman E, Kebe B, Ouedraogo S, Youdeowei A. Enhancing Crop-Livestock Systems in Conservation Agriculture for Sustainable Production Intensification: A Farmer Discovery Process Going to Scale in Burkina Faso. Food and Agriculture Organization of the United Nations (FAO), Integrated Crop Management; 2009;**7**:42. ISSN: 1020-4555. ISBN: 9789251065082

[30] Mutibvu T et al. Constraints and opportunities for increased livestock production in communal areas: A case

study of Simbe, Zimbabwe. Livestock Research for Rural Development. 2012;**24**:9

[31] Welburn SC, Beange I, Ducrotoy MJ, Okello AL. The neglected zoonoses—The case for integrated control and advocacy. Clinical Microbiology and Infection. 2015;**21**(5):433-443. DOI: 10.1016/j.cmi.2015.04.011

[32] Grace D. Food safety in low and middle-income countries. International Journal of Environmental Research and Public Health. 2015;**12**(9):10490-10507. DOI: 10.3390/ijerph120910490

[33] Zinsstag J et al. One Health Theory and Practice of Integrated Health Approach; Switzerland: Swiss Tropical and Public Health Institute; Herston, Australia: University of Queensland; Canada: University of Guelph. 1st edition. March 2015:480. DOI: 10.1079/9781780643410.0000. ISBN-10: 1780643411

Chapter 4

Leptospirosis: Rising Nuisance for Cattle and Threat to Public Health

Amjad Islam Aqib, Muhammad Ijaz, Shahid Hussain Farooqi, Muhammad Shoaib, Muhammad Fakhar-e-Alam Kulyar and Khadija Yasmeen

Abstract

Leptospirosis is a communicable disease at farms that results in abortion and pathological changes in animals and human respectively. Disease is majorly spreading through indirect contact with contaminated urine material. The causative agent belongs to *Leptospira* genus having 21 species, 25 serogroups, and 250 serovars. The prevalence noted at world level is counted to be 41.39% with 30.11% in Asia, 25.62% in Africa, and 46.42% in South Africa. The virulence is attributed to Loa22 protein which is the first protein identified as essential virulence factor. Pathogenesis involves vasculitis following which are direct cytotoxicity and immunological injury resulting in renal failure. Direct examination, PCR, isothermal methods, microscopic agglutination test (MAT) and IgM enzyme-linked immunosorbent assay (ELISA) are diagnostic approaches for leptospirosis. The MAT is a gold standard test for leptospirosis identification. Doxycycline and azithromycin were used as drugs against leptospirosis in mild and severe cases of leptospirosis. Further studies are needed regarding identification, treatment, and effective vaccination.

Keywords: leptospirosis, *Leptospira*, disease outbreaks, leptospirosis vaccine, *Leptospira* tests, epidemiology, prevalence

1. Introduction

Leptospirosis is a worldwide but more neglected zoonotic disease that usually affects humans and animals around the world [1–3] with case records 350,000 annually [4]. Death occurs from 10 to 50% in severe infection cases [5]. Pathogenic *Leptospira* are bacteria that cause the disease through penetration into the mucous membrane or damaged skin of the host [6]and then transfer to the proximal tubule of the kidneys [7]. Infected animals remain asymptomatic and secrete infectious organisms in urine throughout their lifetime [8]. *Leptospira* are excreted in the urine for weeks, months, or longer [9]. It pollutes moist soil, farm land, and rivers. Infection occurs when a person or animal is in intimate contact with a contaminated climate or infected urine of host [6]. The famous *Leptospira* carriers are wild, domestic, and some other mammalian species [10]. Occurrence of leptospirosis in humans is also associated with high temperature, high humidity, and basic hygienic conditions [11, 12]. Human leptospirosis is biphasic, with the general symptoms of pyrogens associated with acute or leptospiremic phase, continuing for about 1 week, and subsequent of

 IntechOpen

recovery or immunization which is defined by antibody production [13]. In the past few decades, leptospirosis has become an infectious disease of urban environments especially in industrialized and developing countries. Rural areas are also affected with high mortality due to delay in diagnosis and lack of infrastructure with adequate clinical suspicion and other unknown causes like inherent pathogenicity of *Leptospira* strains [8]. Leptospirosis is very common in tropical and subtropical areas where people are very close to animals. Warm and humid environment favors in distribution and survival of pathogen [14]. Sporadic cases are reported throughout the year with incidence ranges from 0.1 to 10 per 100,000 people; and during the epidemic, it can reach over 50 per 10,000 people. Most cases are reported in Sri Lanka, India, Indonesia, Maldives, and Thailand. In the past, Sri Lanka (2008), Jakarta (2003), and Mumbai (2005) have been reported as epidemic areas of Southeast Asia [10]. The molecular classification of *Leptospira* in different species is described on DNA correlation base [3, 15]. The genome of *Leptospira* consists of two round chromosomes whose entire sequence has been established recently [8, 16]. The genome is larger than the genomes of other spirochetes, which shows the viability of *Leptospira* in different harsh environments [17]. Symptoms usually appear suddenly after an incubation period of 2–20 days, with a duration of 14 days at least. About 10% of patients diagnosed with leptospirosis having signs like Weil's disease, which manifests itself as jaundice, kidney failure, and hemorrhagic in pulmonary arteries [18]. Leptospirosis is usually related to headache, fever with muscular pain in both adults and children. Drowsiness, vomiting, abdominal pain, diarrhea, cough, photophobia, arthralgia, and constipation may also occur [19].

2. Etiology

Leptospirosis is a prominent communicable disease caused by spirochete bacteria. The bacterial species belong to genus *Leptospira* that have ability to cause a disease in a variety of wild and domestic animal bases [3]. Spirochetes bacteria are motile having hook form or question-mark shape and range in size from 6 to 20 μm in length and 0.1 μm in thickness [4]. Family Leptospiraceae includes genus *Leptospira*, which is further divided into two strains, that is, pathogenic and saprophytic [4, 15]. Pathogenic *Leptospira* have 21 species, 25 serogroups, and 250 serovars [3, 5]. *Leptospira* spp. are obligate aerobes having sluggish growth. Ideal growth temperature for *Leptospira* is 28–30°C [16]. There are different other characteristics of *Leptospira* like size, number of genes and pseudogenes, etc. (**Figure 1**). Serovars "pomona and grippotyphosa" are expectedly found to be the most prevalent candidates [17]. Leptospirosis in cattle is caused by *Leptospira borgpetersenii* and *Leptospira interrogans* serovar Hardjo, strains (well adapted to cattle) Hardjo bovis and Hardjo prajitno [18]. In Brazil as well as in Latin America, L. borgpetersenii serovar Hardjo strain Hardjo bovis were isolated from naturally infected cattle. Before this study, only serological studies had shown reactive animals with the serovar Hardjo in various countries [20, 21]. In Brazil, Chile, England, and Columbia, serovar Hardjo was found most prevalent among cattle [22]. Between 1988 and 2007 in France, serovar Serjoe (34%) was most common in cattle [23]. There are different reservoir hosts of *Leptospira* (**Table 1**).

2.1 Prevalence of leptospirosis

Worldwide, the prevalence of animal leptospirosis is reported between 2 and 46% depending upon animal species [12]. More than 15 serogroups of *Leptospira* is observed and isolated from cattle, for example, icterohaemorrhagiae, canicola, pomona and grippotyphosa, etc. (Rocha). Seroprevalence of different serovars is different in all countries or regions. *L. bratislava* and *L. grippotyphosa* are more in Spain in those cattle which do not have good reproductive health [21]. Latin American countries, like Venezuela, have high prevalence of leptospirosis (80.51%) along with predominance of Sejroe serovar. Lesser incidence (2.6%) of disease has been observed in Peru during desiccated season when there are less chances for bacterial survival and transmission [24]. Similar results have been observed in Colombia and Mexico with the prevalence of 16.4–60.9% and 28.4–52%, respectively [25, 26]. Particularly, in countries like India, the bovine leptospirosis is highly

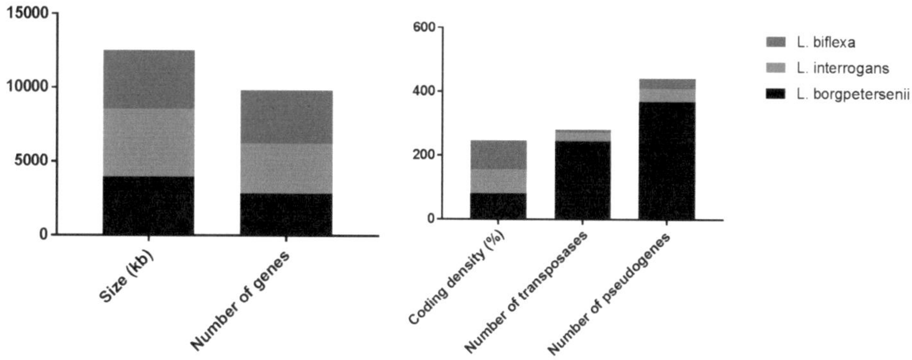

Figure 1.
Main characteristics of pathogenic and trophic genome Leptospira spp. [20].

Reservoir host	Serovar	Reference
Pigs	Pomona, Tarassovi	[8]
Cattle	Hardjo, Pomona	
Horse	Bratislava	
Dog	Canicola	
Sheep	Hardjo	
Rats	Icterohaemorrhagiae, Copenhageni	
Bats	Cynopteri, Wolffi	

Table 1.
Typical reservoir hosts of Leptospira.

Country	Year	Diagnostic methods	Specie	Prevalence%	Reference
India	1983 2011	— MAT	Cattle —	68 87	[35] [36]
Malaysia	1987	MAT	Cattle Buffalo	40.5 31	[37]
Sri Lanka	2011 2014	MAT Nested PCR	Cattle Cattle	20.31 12.2	[38] [6]
Iran	2011	MAT	Cattle	19.10	[39]
Pakistan	2018	Indirect ELISA	Cattle Buffalo	25.52 20.72	[40]
Bangladesh	2015	ELISA	Cattle	47.27	[41]

Table 2.
Prevalence of bovine leptospirosis in different countries of Asia.

prevalent, that is, up to 87% [27], 89.9% in Poland, and 88.2% in Mexico [28]. In contrary, certain states present lesser incidence, for example, 31.3% in Brazil [29], 27.4% in Australia [30], 30.3% in Tanzania [31], 20.3% in Sri Lanka [32], and 19.1% in Iran [33] (**Table 2**). These variations could be due to altered topographical localities, husbandry and farm management applications, infection immunity among diverse rears, and intensities of normal resistance [29]. In urban areas, leptospirosis is broadly prevalent, as stated by Platts-Mills [34].

3. Pathogenesis

Leptospirosis is termed as "storm of abortion" and is farm economy jeopardizing malaise [42]. *Leptospira* spread in direct and indirect ways, while the latter is a more pronounced method of transfer. Direct transmission involves through infected urine, post abortion uterine discharge, sexual contact, and infected placentae. Indirect involves contact with environment. Bacteria get entry to skin through abraded skin that follows hematogenous spread in the body. Bacteria result vasculitis that in turn results into either direct cytotoxic injury and immunological reactions or massive migration of fluid from intravascular to interstitial compartment. The latter results in renal dysfunction and vascular injury to internal organs. Pathogenic *Leptospira* could not be phagocytosed by macrophages and neutrophils, but if there are specific antibodies present, it can be phagocytosed [22]. It has been suggested that the animals are susceptible to severe or acute leptospirosis caused by increase in production of anti-inflammatory cytokines and chemokines [23]. Although pathogenic *Leptospira* are complementary to bactericidal activity, it has long been known that *Leptospira* has antimicrobial activity [43]. In most studies, leptospiral proteins that bind to one or more components are usually identified in recombinant form. Adhesin LenA (LfhA, Lsa 24) and Len B also bind to complementary regulatory protein factor H [44, 45]. Complement resistance to pathogenic *Leptospira* can also bind to the complement module C4BP, which catalyzes the cleavage of C4b [24]. It leads to decrease in surface deposition of subsequent components of the complement, where decaying species are not available. In subsequent studies, this activity was attributed to the new leptospiral proteins LcpA and Lsa30 [46]. Interestingly, ligand proteins that interact with many host ECM hosts and other proteins also interact with the complement regulators H, FHL-1, FHR1, and C4BP [25]. Surprisingly, the *Leptospira* elongation factor Tu shows a superficial effect and interaction with factor H, as well as binding to many purified host proteins, which leads to its diversity, the so-called "moonlighting protein" [25]. Most of the above studies provide indirect evidence of the role of *Leptospira* protein in the prevention of complement, but recently, it has been shown that the pathogenicity and non-urogenital fecundity of the three complement pathways, including factor B [26]. C2 and C4b are identified in the culture supernatant of the *Leptospira* cleavage component. In fact, inactivation of the above two proteins, Lig B and Len B, does not have a significant effect on pathogenicity [27, 28, 47]. Similarly, functional redundancy must also be considered: LenA and LenB. All proteins have structural and functional similarities to the endostatin of mammals [44].

3.1 Known virulence factors

The emergence of the mutagenesis system revealed a small number of *Leptospira* genes that encode the components necessary for the manifestation of pathogenicity. The first leptospiral protein, identified as virulence, is Loa 22, and the outer membrane protein containing the C-terminal OmpA domain appears to mediate the connection between the outer membrane and the peptidoglycan layer (mutant hama loa 22). The presence of a homolog of Loa 22 in *L. biflexa* has an indirect effect on pathogenicity. Since lipopolysaccharide (LPS) is a pathogenic factor for all Gram-negative bacteria, it is not surprising that this hypothesis cannot be obtained until a certain mutant is identified in the *Leptospira*, studies eliminate motility by inactivating flagellated structures or genes involved in biosynthesis. Inactivation of fliY-encoding choleretic switching protein reduces toxicity in guinea pigs [29]. Mutations in the gene encoding the sensory protein LB139 reduce motility and down-regulation of a number of chemotactic genes and weaken the mutant for hamsters [30]. The lack of similar genes in vegetative bacilli strongly suggests the survival of mammalian species as well as in nutrition intake. Indeed, studies have shown toxicity related activities of *Leptospira* sphingomyelinase such as pore formation and cytotoxicity [31]. However, the key role of leptospiral sphingomyelinase in the pathogenesis is not genetically established. Recently, it has been shown that *Leptospira*-LruA [48] plays an important role in autoimmune response, which is associated with mammalian apolipoprotein A1 [49].

4. Transmission

Transmission of *Leptospira* occurs often with direct contact with infected urine, placenta, or milk. Transmission through venereal or transplacental route is also possible, whereas the most common route is infected urine. If there are leptospiral infected animals present in a dairy farm, the environment is also contaminated. Dairy feeder calves are probably the largest carriers of *Leptospira* in commercial feed yards. Dairy calves have the habit of sucking the scrotum of other calves in the pen, so this would be direct contamination of infected urine from carriers by suckling habit. *Leptospira* survives in the moist, damp, and moderately warm environment and can be easily killed by freezing, dehydration, and direct sunlight (**Figure 2**).

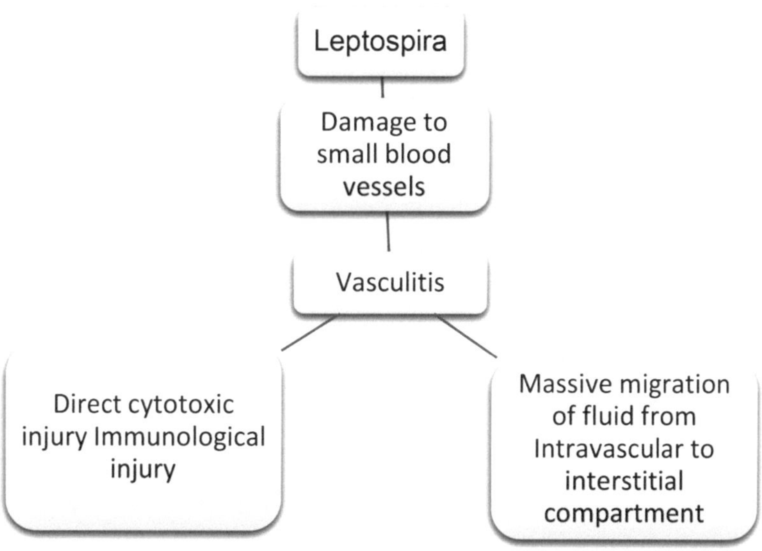

Figure 2.
Mechanism of Leptospira.

5. Diagnosis

Infection occurred by pathogenic leptospires is divided into two stages, first stage is acute stage or septicaemia (because septicaemia is in this stage), which lasts from 7 to 10 days with headache and myalgia. The second stage is immune stage which is after first week of infection and lasts 4–30 days [34]. During first stage, leptospires are present in blood and can say bacterial count is high in the blood, while when second stage starts, then the level of antibodies IgM and IgG start to increase and this increase in antibodies titer is correlated to elimination of leptospires from blood. *Leptospira* antigens and DNA sometimes may not be detected from the blood; this may be due to late sampling, or sampling in acute stage where proper level of leptospiremia is not developed and due to antibiotic administration, leptospires are eliminated from the blood. False negative results will be there, if we detect antibodies prior to sero-conversion during acute stage. Coagulated blood has serum and clot while non-coagulated blood has plasma, RBCs, WBCs and platelets. That can be collected according to the tests. If you are going to do gene amplification than EDTA, plasma gives the best results [50]. Leptospires can be detected in urine and cerebrospinal fluid samples. Many kits are available in the market for rapid detection of leptospires from blood, urine, and CSF sample; these kits basically detect nucleic acid of leptospires, but for these tests, purification of nucleic acid is required [51].

5.1 Current tools and emerging technologies for diagnosis of *Leptospira*

Different tools are being developed for the study of virulence factors, pathogenicity, and basic cell biology of organisms [52]. These are essential for proper treatment and reduction of the severity of the disease. During acute infection, nonspecific symptoms of leptospires mimic the febrile condition, which are essential for proper treatment and reduce the severity of the disease. Therefore, the diagnosis of leptospirosis is highly dependent on the particular laboratory tests [13]. Serology is the dominant one in diagnosis, while the micro-aggregation test (MAT) is the standard serological reference method. MAT is a sensitive test due to the antigenic heterogeneity of *Leptospira*, which require a large number of serovars as antigens. Furthermore, it is useless at early stage of the disease when antibodies are not present or present in less quantity [18]. Detection of disease in early stage helps the epidemiological investigators. However, antigen detection at this stage is more expensive and complex [13]. Current diagnostic tools for *Leptospira* detections other than MAT are rapid antibody-based tests, direct examination of blood, the rapid nucleic-acid diagnosis, [53], dark field microscopy (DFM), IgM ELISA, and polymerase chain reaction (PCR) [13].

5.1.1 Direct examination

This method is cheap, but for direct examination, dark field microscope is required [54]. Theoretically, leptospires may be diagnosed by direct examination of blood during first week after onset of symptoms. Leptospires are 6–20 μm long and their diameter is 0.15 μm. Because of their size, dark field microscopy is required; 10^{-2}–10^{-6} leptospires/mL of blood may be observed during the acute stage of leptospirosis [55].

5.1.2 Gene amplification

5.1.2.1 PCR

The use of PCR is increasing in recent years and it has replaced the serological methods in endemic areas, because it is more sensitive and has capacity to give early diagnosis. Real-time PCR is faster than regular PCR [56]. The threshold level in the urine or blood is 10–100 leptospires/mL (**Figures 3** and **4**) [50, 57].

5.1.2.2 Isothermal methods

In recent years, many isothermal amplification techniques are developed like isothermal technique [59]. This technique can be used as alternative to the PCR. There is no need for constant maintenance of temperature at 60–65°C and no thermal recycler is required; so, these things make it best for developing countries.

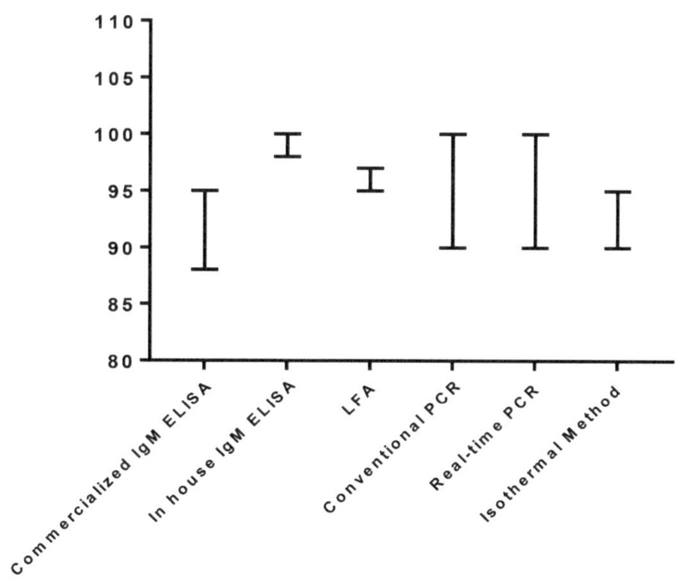

Figure 3.
Specificity of different diagnostic tests during acute phase of leptospirosis [56, 58].

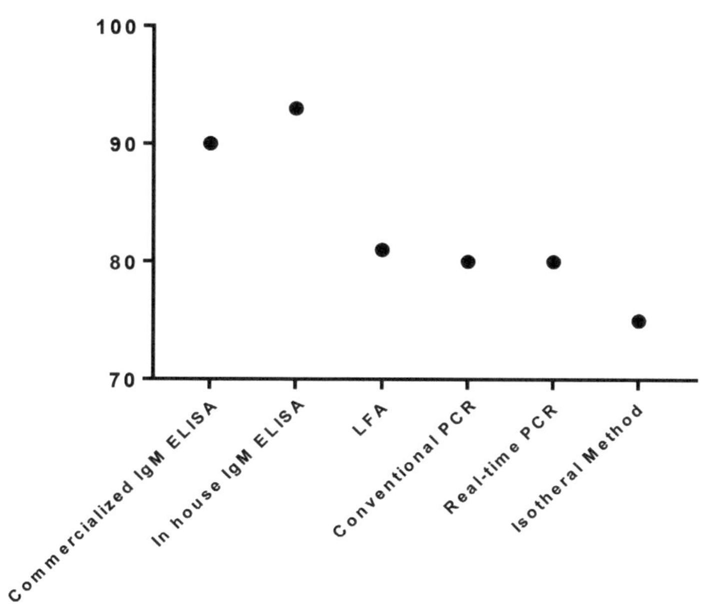

Figure 4.
Sensitivity of different diagnostic tests during acute phase of leptospirosis [58].

For this, an effective and specific amplification is performed by DNA polymerase and six primers in 1 hour under isothermal conditions. Now the amplified DNA can be easily detected by eye observation of fluorescence without using gel electrophoresis [60]. Loop-mediated isothermal amplification (LAMP) methods are recently developed for the quick diagnosis of pathogenic leptospires, and lipL41 and rrs are the genes targeted by LAMP. The specificity of these methods is weak because these can detect the threshold between 2 and 100 leptospires/reactive mixture [61].

5.1.3 Serological tests

5.1.3.1 The microscopic agglutination test (MAT)

This microscopic agglutination test is developed in Pasteur Institute. Dark field microscopy is required to see agglutination of live leptospires cultures with patient's serum. This is the gold standard test for leptospirosis. It determines the anti-*Leptospira* immunoglobulin titers in human and animal serum at the serogroup level, so it is used for clinical and epidemiological investigations [62]. MAT is performed on micro titration plates, dilutions of serum which is collected from the patient is made and then equal volume of leptospiral culture is added to form agglutinations of distinctive patterns that consist of highly dense packs of partly intact leptospires. The test is read by DFM.

5.1.3.2 IgM enzyme-linked immunosorbent assay (ELISA)

Normal ELISA is commonly used to diagnose leptospirosis. Enzyme immunoassay of leptospirosis can be performed using a commercially available kit or antigen obtained internally. Which is commonly used to detect IgM, and sometimes to detect IgG antibodies against leptospiral antigens. The presence of IgM antibodies indicates current or recent leptospirosis. The commercially available *Leptospira* IgM ELISA is used for the serological detection of acute leptospirosis infection in a patient's serum sample. This ELISA is based on the principle that any *Leptospira* IgM antibody present in the patient's serum binds to the *Leptospira* antigen that adheres to the microporous surface of the microwell. Residual serum was removed from these wells by washing with 1% buffer (included in the kit). Peroxidase-conjugated anti-human IgM is presented after adding to the wells, and the plate is reincubated so that the bound antigen-antibody complex binds to the conjugate. The wells are washed again and a colorless substrate system, tetramethylbenzidine hydroperoxide, is added. The substrate is hydrolyzed, and the chromogen is blue. When the reaction is stopped with phosphoric acid, TMB turns yellow. The development of color indicates the presence of visual acuity IgM antibody against *Leptospira* in serum samples [63].

6. Necropsy findings

Cows with acute leptospirosis are characterized by anemia, jaundice, hemoglobinuria, and lower lobe hemorrhage. An ulcer and bleeding may be present on the mucous membrane of the peritoneum. Pulmonary edema and emphysema are also common in cattle. Histologically, there is a progressive and diffuse interstitial nephritis and liver necrosis in the centre of the lobules. Sometimes the vascular lesions of the meninges are transferred to chronic infections. *Leptospira* can be seen in the silvery spots of a part of tortuous tubules proximal to the kidneys. In acute infection, there is minimal inflammation, and in the middle of the leaflet, there are only tubes filled with hemoglobin and visible liver necrosis. At a later stage, progressive interstitial nephritis is characterized by a small white cortical lesion, which initially slightly increases or decreases with increasing age of the lesion. The fruit of a broken cow is usually automated by the fact that there is no damage or bacteria. Even fresh fruit, positive identification of leptospirosis in lesions is not easy. Although the use of fluorescent antibody technology facilitates the identification of organisms, false positive results are common unless experienced diagnosticians interpret the test. Although dark field microscopy can be attempted, it is not suitable for tissue collected at dissection. Although PCR technology is important, in some cases, several primer sequences may be required.

Samples for confirmation of diagnosis are kidney, liver and placenta. Histology of kidney, liver, brain, heart, lungs and placenta can be performed. While for serological analysis heart blood serum or pericardial fluid from foetus can also be obtained.

The zoonotic potential of this organism should keep in mind during handling of carcasses and submitting specimens.

7. Treatment

Treatment is based on severity of illness being presented by animal which in most of the cases is mild and self-limiting requiring no care. Other considerations, while treatment is considered, include differential diagnosis, cost, and availability of drugs. Treatment obtained based on in-vitro studies presented doxycycline, ampicillin, azithromycin or amoxicillin [64]. The double-blind randomized trials conducted on 29 patients produced promising results by reducing symptoms of malaise in 2 days preventing leptospiremia. The treatment, however, was not conclusive prevention from progression to severity [65]. Doxycycline or azithromycin is the drug of choice in endemic areas while contraindicated in pregnancy [64]. Sever cases are responsive to penicillin G sodium in studies conducted before 90s. The emerging resistance has narrowed spectrum of antibiotic use against infections [66]. Open randomized trial conducted with experiment involving 256 patients proved nonsignificant difference among penicillin G, cefotaxime, and doxycycline antibiotics [67]. Some of meta-analysis studies have reported nonsignificant difference between penicillin G and placebo on mortality [68]. Mortality is reported to increase up to 70% with pulmonary involvement which is due to immune-mediated inflammatory response. The therapeutic indicated for this complication is steroidal drugs. Early steroid administration was found responsive but methodologically flawed in various studies. Desmopressin was evaluated in various randomized studies as adjunct therapy with nonsignificant mortality benefits [69]. Therapy is considered beneficial with doxycycline or azithromycin along with steroid administration in mild and severe cases. Variations in studies are reported with nonsignificant benefits to mortality reduction.

7.1 Blood transfusion

Leptospirosis is a zoonosis with worldwide distribution. It is more prevalent in the developing countries. Hemorrhagic manifestations constitute the common clinical feature in leptospirosis [70]. In cattle, acute hemolytic syndrome of leptospirosis has been reported characterized by fever, icterus, anemia, and hemoglobinuria [71]. Without effective treatment, hemolytic syndrome in cattle may result in death. A high mortality rate of severe disease was determined to be associated with certain serotypes of *Leptospira* [72]. The disease, for instance, causes a decrease in erythrocyte and platelet counts, leading to anemia and hemorrhagic diathesis, respectively.

Elevated bilirubin levels result from hemolysis and hepatorenal failure, indicating the characteristic nature of clinical signs [73]. Blood transfusion was reported to be quite effective in cases of life-threatening anemia in cattle. Previous reports suggest that timely transfusion of whole fresh blood be administrated to overcome severe hemolytic leptospirosis. Indeed, transfusion providing the vital components such as erythrocytes, platelets, and plasma contributes to repair the present collapses, that is, anemia, hemorrhagic diathesis, septicemia, and hepatorenal failure, in affected cattle [71]. A PCV value of 15% or less developing acutely may require transfusion, while chronic anemia can be tolerated in cattle without any transfusion [74].

7.2 Vaccination

The optimal control regime for leptospirosis is to prevent clinical disease and exfoliation in the urine in animals exposed to different serotypes of *Leptospira*. The most common method of controlling leptospirosis in cattle is vaccination and selective treatment. In addition, proper quarantine procedures should be implemented to prevent the introduction of hajo in the herd by buying infected animals. However, leptospirosis and wild animals gave rise as a carrier of the prevalence of serotypes of hardjo infections in cattle, mainly to prevent the overall impact of leptospirosis in most dairy products and Rieben beef failure. This is impossible. Thus, vaccination depends on an increase in the resistance of an animal to leptospiral serotype infection in this area. In all cases, the effort (buildings, under the control of rodents around swamps and creeks, for example, surround) must be made in order to limit direct and indirect contact between the cattle and Leptospirosetragern. In addition, proper quarantine procedures should be implemented to prevent the introduction of hajo in the herd by buying infected animals. However, leptospirosis and wild animals gave rise as a carrier of the prevalence of serotypes of hardjo infections in cattle, mainly to prevent the overall impact of leptospirosis in most dairy products and Rieben beef failure. This is impossible. Thus, vaccination depends on an increase in the resistance of an animal to leptospiral serotype infection in this area. The leptoral vaccine currently available for cattle in the United States is a 5-fold bacterial whole cell vaccine, including Pomona, Canicola, Icterohaemorrhagiae, Grippotyphosa, and Hardjo serotypes. These antigens can also be used in various combinations of other viral and bacterial vaccines. In the United States, a series of experimental studies and field data are available from the United States. Typical leptospirosis vaccines are Hajo kidney serotype infection, urinary tract infection or fetus (ha-ha type). This does not exclude the fact that the state indicates that the country is isolated from the United States. Many of the available Hardjo vaccines were approved many years ago in rigorous efficacy studies that mimic the natural route of exposure, and the last method to determine whether the Hardjo serotypes are infected with cattle is Hardjo stocks which did not use the serotype. However, recently two Hardjo vaccine serotypes have been widely studied using appropriate strains and methods. Compared to many other Hardjo serotype vaccines, these two products have shown excellent protection against infection and Hardjo hemoglobin isolation [75].

8. Conclusion

Leptospirosis is a major zoonotic disease resulting in high mortality in humans and animals. The disease is diagnosed clinically by fever, headache, vomiting, abdominal pain, and arthralgia. Leptospirosis is caused by more than 250 serovars, while pomona and grippotyphosa being the most prevalent serovars among them. However, among cattle, serovar Hardjo is the most important in causation of disease. Among the Asian countries, the highest prevalence of leptospirosis was found in India. Leptospirosis is mainly transmitted by direct contact with infected urine, and bacteria are mainly entered through ruptured skin. In house IgM ELISA is highly specific technique for *Leptospira* diagnosis. However, among the serological test, ELISA is more sensitive test for *Leptospira* diagnosis. Most effective treatment for *Leptospira* is doxycycline or azithromycin; however, former is not recommended in pregnancy. However, in severe cases, blood transfusion is also a best choice to save the life of animal. At last, the most effective way to control the disease is vaccination at early age of life following booster doses to avoid from more severe economic losses.

Author details

Amjad Islam Aqib[1*], Muhammad Ijaz[2], Shahid Hussain Farooqi[3], Muhammad Shoaib[4], Muhammad Fakhar-e-Alam Kulyar[5] and Khadija Yasmeen[5]

1 Department of Medicine, Cholistan University of Veterinary and Animal Sciences, Bahawalpur, Pakistan

2 Department of Clinical Medicine and Surgery, University of Veterinary and Animal Sciences, Lahore, Pakistan

3 Department of Clinical Sciences, KBCMA College of Veterianary and Animal Sciences, Narowal, Pakistan

4 Institute of Microbiology, University of Agriculture, Faisalabad, Pakistan

5 Department of Clinical Medicine and Surgery, Faculty of Veterinary Sciences, University of Agriculture, Faisalabad, Pakistan

*Address all correspondence to: amjadwaseer@gmail.com

IntechOpen

© 2019 The Author(s). Licensee IntechOpen. This chapter is distributed under the terms of the Creative Commons Attribution License (http://creativecommons.org/licenses/by/3.0), which permits unrestricted use, distribution, and reproduction in any medium, provided the original work is properly cited. (cc) BY

References

[1] Costa F, Hagan JE, Calcagno J, Kane M, Torgerson P, Martinez-Silveira MS, et al. Global morbidity and mortality of leptospirosis: A systematic review. PLoS Neglected Tropical Diseases. 2015;**9**(9):e0003898

[2] Lambert A, Takahashi N, Charon N, Picardeau M. Chemotactic behavior of pathogenic and non-pathogenic Leptospira species. Applied and Environmental Microbiology. 2012;**78**(23):8467-8469

[3] Brenner DJ, Kaufmann AF, Sulzer KR, Steigerwalt AG, Rogers FC, Weyant RS. Further determination of DNA relatedness between serogroups and serovars in the family Leptospiraceae with a proposal for Leptospira alexanderi sp. nov. and four new Leptospira genomospecies. International Journal of Systematic and Evolutionary Microbiology. 1999;**49**(2):839-858

[4] Terpstra W. Human Leptospirosis: Guidance for Diagnosis, Surveillance and Control. World Health Organization; 2003

[5] Marchiori E, Lourenço S, Setúbal S, Zanetti G, Gasparetto TD, Hochhegger B. Clinical and imaging manifestations of hemorrhagic pulmonary leptospirosis: A state-of-the-art review. Lung. 2011;**189**(1):1-9

[6] Gamage CD, Koizumi N, Perera AC, Muto M, Nwafor-Okoli C, Ranasinghe S, et al. Carrier status of leptospirosis among cattle in Sri Lanka: A zoonotic threat to public health. Transboundary and Emerging Diseases. 2014;**61**(1):91-96

[7] Athanazio DA, Silva EF, Santos CS, Rocha GM, Vannier-Santos MA, McBride AJ, et al. Rattus norvegicus as a model for persistent renal colonization by pathogenic Leptospira interrogans. Acta Tropica. 2008;**105**(2):176-180

[8] Bharti AR, Nally JE, Ricaldi JN, Matthias MA, Diaz MM, Lovett MA, et al. Leptospirosis: A zoonotic disease of global importance. The Lancet Infectious Diseases. 2003;**3**(12):757-771

[9] Sejvar J, Bancroft E, Winthrop K, Bettinger J, Bajani M, Bragg S, et al. Leptospirosis in "eco-challenge" athletes, Malaysian Borneo, 2000. Emerging Infectious Diseases. 2003;**9**(6):702

[10] Tique V, Mattar S, Miranda J, Oviedo M, Noda A, Montes E, Rodriguez V. Clinical and Epidemiological Status of Leptospirosis in a Tropical Caribbean Area of Colombia. BioMed research international. 2018;**2018**

[11] Lau CL, Smythe LD, Craig SB, Weinstein P. Climate change, flooding, urbanisation and leptospirosis: Fuelling the fire? Transactions of the Royal Society of Tropical Medicine and Hygiene. 2010;**104**(10):631-638

[12] Ricaldi JN, Vinetz JM. Leptospirosis in the tropics and in travelers. Current Infectious Disease Reports. 2006;**8**(1):51-58

[13] Schreier S, Doungchawee G, Chadsuthi S, Triampo D, Triampo W. Leptospirosis: Current situation and trends of specific laboratory tests. Expert Review of Clinical Immunology. 2013;**9**(3):263-280

[14] Hartskeerl R, Collares-Pereira M, Ellis W. Emergence, control and re-emerging leptospirosis: Dynamics of infection in the changing world. Clinical Microbiology and Infection. 2011;**17**(4):494-501

[15] Perolat P, Chappel R, Adler B, Baranton G, Bulach D, Billinghurst M,

et al. Leptospira fainei sp. nov., isolated from pigs in Australia. International Journal of Systematic and Evolutionary Microbiology. 1998;**48**(3):851-858

[16] Ren S-X, Fu G, Jiang X-G, Zeng R, Miao Y-G, Xu H, et al. Unique physiological and pathogenic features of Leptospira interrogans revealed by whole-genome sequencing. Nature. 2003;**422**(6934):888

[17] de la Peña-Moctezuma A, Bulach DM, Kalambaheti T, Adler B. Comparative analysis of the LPS biosynthetic loci of the genetic subtypes of serovar Hardjo: Leptospira interrogans subtype Hardjoprajitno and Leptospira borgpetersenii subtype Hardjobovis. FEMS Microbiology Letters. 1999;**177**(2):319-326

[18] Budihal SV, Perwez K. Leptospirosis diagnosis: Competancy of various laboratory tests. Journal of Clinical and Diagnostic Research: JCDR. 2014;**8**(1):199

[19] Haake DA, Levett PN. Leptospirosis in humans. Current Topics in Microbiology and Immunology. 2015;**387**:65-97

[20] Adler B, de la Peña Moctezuma A. Leptospira and leptospirosis. Veterinary Microbiology. 2010;**140**(3-4):287-296

[21] Guitian F, García-Peña F, Oliveira J, Sanjuan M, Yus E. Serological study of the frequency of leptospiral infections among dairy cows in farms with suboptimal reproductive efficiency in Galicia, Spain. Veterinary Microbiology. 2001;**80**(3):275-284

[22] Ko AI, Goarant C, Picardeau M. Leptospira: The dawn of the molecular genetics era for an emerging zoonotic pathogen. Nature Reviews Microbiology. 2009;**7**(10):736

[23] Matsui M, Rouleau V, Bruyère-Ostells L, Goarant C. Gene expression profiles of immune mediators and histopathological findings in animal models of leptospirosis: Comparison between susceptible hamsters and resistant mice. Infection and Immunity. 2011;**79**(11):4480-4492

[24] Barbosa AS, Abreu PA, Vasconcellos SA, Morais ZM, Gonçales AP, Silva AS, et al. Immune evasion of leptospira species by acquisition of human complement regulator C4BP. Infection and Immunity. 2009;**77**(3):1137-1143

[25] Wolff DG, Castiblanco-Valencia MM, Abe CM, Monaris D, Morais ZM, Souza GO, et al. Interaction of leptospira elongation factor Tu with plasminogen and complement factor H: A metabolic leptospiral protein with moonlighting activities. PLoS One. 2013;**8**(11):e81818

[26] Fraga TR, Courrol DS, Castiblanco-Valencia MM, Hirata IY, Vasconcellos SA, Juliano L, et al. Immune evasion by pathogenic leptospira strains: The secretion of proteases that directly cleave complement proteins. The Journal of Infectious Diseases. 2013;**209**(6):876-886

[27] Adler B, Lo M, Seemann T, Murray GL. Pathogenesis of leptospirosis: The influence of genomics. Veterinary Microbiology. 2011;**153**(1-2):73-81

[28] Murray GL, Srikram A, Henry R, Puapairoj A, Sermswan RW, Adler B. Leptospira interrogans requires heme oxygenase for disease pathogenesis. Microbes and Infection. 2009;**11**(2):311-314

[29] Liao S, Sun A, Ojcius DM, Wu S, Zhao J, Yan J. Inactivation of the fliY gene encoding a flagellar motor switch protein attenuates mobility and virulence of leptospira interrogans strain Lai. BMC Microbiology. 2009;**9**(1):253

[30] Eshghi A, Becam J, Lambert A, Sismeiro O, Dillies MA, Jagla B, et al.

A putative regulatory genetic locus modulates virulence in the pathogen Leptospira interrogans. Infection and Immunity. 2014;**82**(6):2542-2552

[31] Lee SH, Kim S, Park SC, Kim MJ. Cytotoxic activities of Leptospira interrogans hemolysin SphH as a pore-forming protein on mammalian cells. Infection and Immunity. 2002;**70**(1):315-322

[32] Markey B, Leonard F, Archambault M, Cullinane A, Maguire D. Clinical Veterinary Microbiology E-Book. Elsevier Health Sciences; 2013

[33] Boonsilp S, Thaipadungpanit J, Amornchai P, Wuthiekanun V, Bailey MS, Holden MT, et al. A single multilocus sequence typing (MLST) scheme for seven pathogenic Leptospira species. PLoS Neglected Tropical Diseases. 2013;**7**(1):e1954

[34] Picardeau M. Diagnosis and epidemiology of leptospirosis. Médecine et Maladies Infectieuses. 2013;**43**(1):1-9

[35] Ratnam S, Sundararaj T, Subramanian S. Serological evidence of leptospirosis in a human population following an outbreak of the disease in cattle. Transactions of the Royal Society of Tropical Medicine and Hygiene. 1983;**77**(1):94-98

[36] Natarajaseenivasan K, Vedhagiri K, Sivabalan V, Prabagaran SG, Sukumar S, Artiushin SC, et al. Seroprevalence of Leptospira borgpetersenii serovar javanica infection among dairy cattle, rats and humans in the Cauvery river valley of southern India. Southeast Asian Journal of Tropical Medicine and Public Health. 2011;**42**(3):679

[37] Bahaman A, Ibrahim A, Adam H. Serological prevalence of leptospiral infection in domestic animals in West Malaysia. Epidemiology and Infection. 1987;**99**(2):379-392

[38] Gamage CD, Koizumi N, Muto M, Nwafor-Okoli C, Kurukurusuriya S, Rajapakse JR, et al. Prevalence and carrier status of leptospirosis in smallholder dairy cattle and peridomestic rodents in Kandy, Sri Lanka. Vector Borne and Zoonotic Diseases. 2011;**11**(8):1041-1047

[39] Tabatabaeizadeh E, Tabar GH, Farzaneh N, Seifi HA. Prevalence of Leptospira hardjo antibody in bulk tank milk in some dairy herds in Mashhad suburb. African Journal of Microbiology Research. 2011;**5**(14):1768-1772

[40] Ijaz M, Farooqi SH, Aqib AI, Bakht P, Ali A, Ghaffar A, et al. Sero-epidemiology of bovine leptospirosis and associated risk factors in a flood affected zone of Pakistan. Pakistan Veterinary Journal. 2018;**38**(2):179-183

[41] Parvez M, Prodhan M, Rahman M, Faruque M. Seroprevalence and associated risk factors of Leptospira interrogans serovar Hardjo in dairy cattle of Chittagong, Banladesh. Pakistan Veterinary Journal. 2015;**35**(3):350-354

[42] Ellis WA. Animal leptospirosis. In: Leptospira and leptospirosis. Berlin, Heidelberg: Springer; 2015. pp. 99-137

[43] Zuerner RL. Host response to Leptospira infection. In: Leptospira and Leptospirosis. Springer; 2015. pp. 223-250

[44] Stevenson B, Choy HA, Pinne M, Rotondi ML, Miller MC, DeMoll E, et al. Leptospira interrogans endostatin-like outer membrane proteins bind host fibronectin, laminin and regulators of complement. PLoS One. 2007;**2**(11):e1188

[45] Verma A, Hellwage J, Artiushin S, Zipfel PF, Kraiczy P, Timoney JF, et al. LfhA, a novel factor H-binding protein of Leptospira interrogans. Infection and Immunity. 2006;**74**(5):2659-2666

[46] Souza NM, Vieira ML, Alves IJ, de Morais ZM, Vasconcellos SA, Nascimento AL. Lsa30, a novel adhesin of Leptospira interrogans binds human plasminogen and the complement regulator C4bp. Microbial Pathogenesis. 2012;**53**(3-4):125-134

[47] Croda J, Figueira CP, Wunder EA, Santos CS, Reis MG, Ko AI, et al. Targeted mutagenesis in pathogenic Leptospira species: Disruption of the LigB gene does not affect virulence in animal models of leptospirosis. Infection and Immunity. 2008;**76**(12):5826-5833

[48] Verma A, Stevenson B, Adler B. Leptospirosis in horses. Veterinary Microbiology. 2013;**167**(1-2):61-66

[49] Boonsilp S, Thaipadungpanit J, Amornchai P, Wuthiekanun V, Bailey M. A single multilocus sequence typing (MLST) scheme for seven. 2013

[50] Smythe LD, Smith IL, Smith GA, Dohnt MF, Symonds ML, Barnett LJ, et al. A quantitative PCR (TaqMan) assay for pathogenic *Leptospira* spp. BMC Infectious Diseases. 2002;**2**(1):13

[51] Bourhy P, Bremont S, Zinini F, Giry C, Picardeau M. Comparison of real-time PCR assays for the detection of pathogenic *Leptospira* spp. in blood and identification of variations in target sequences. Journal of Clinical Microbiology. 2011;**49**(6):2154-2160

[52] Saint Girons I, Bourhy P, Ottone C, Picardeau M, Yelton D, Hendrix RW, et al. The LE1 bacteriophage replicates as a plasmid within *Leptospira biflexa*: Construction of an *L. biflexa-Escherichia coli* shuttle vector. Journal of Bacteriology. 2000;**182**(20):5700-5705

[53] Picardeau M, Bertherat E, Jancloes M, Skouloudis AN, Durski K, Hartskeerl RA. Rapid tests for diagnosis of leptospirosis: Current tools and emerging technologies. Diagnostic Microbiology and Infectious Disease. 2014;**78**(1):1-8

[54] Vijayachari P, Sugunan A, Umapathi T, Sehgal S. Evaluation of darkground microscopy as a rapid diagnosis procedure in leptospirosis. Indian Journal of Medical Research. 2001;**114**:54

[55] Agampodi SB, Matthias MA, Moreno AC, Vinetz JM. Utility of quantitative polymerase chain reaction in leptospirosis diagnosis: Association of level of leptospiremia and clinical manifestations in Sri Lanka. Clinical Infectious Diseases. 2012;**54**(9):1249-1255

[56] Ahmed A, Engelberts MF, Boer KR, Ahmed N, Hartskeerl RA. Development and validation of a real-time PCR for detection of pathogenic *Leptospira* species in clinical materials. PLoS One. 2009;**4**(9):e7093

[57] Stoddard RA, Gee JE, Wilkins PP, McCaustland K, Hoffmaster AR. Detection of pathogenic *Leptospira* spp. through TaqMan polymerase chain reaction targeting the LipL32 gene. Diagnostic Microbiology and Infectious Disease. 2009;**64**(3):247-255

[58] Hashimoto VY, Dias JA, Spohr KA, Silva MC, Andrade MG, Müller EE, et al. Prevalência e fatores de risco associados à *Leptospira* spp. em rebanhos bovinos da região centro-sul do estado do Paraná. Embrapa Rondônia-Artigo em periódico indexado (ALICE). 2012

[59] Sonthayanon P, Chierakul W, Wuthiekanun V, Thaipadungpanit J, Kalambaheti T, Boonsilp S, et al. Accuracy of loop-mediated isothermal amplification for diagnosis of human leptospirosis in Thailand. The American Journal of Tropical Medicine and Hygiene. 2011;**84**(4):614-620

[60] Mori Y, Notomi T. Loop-mediated isothermal amplification (LAMP):

A rapid, accurate, and cost-effective diagnostic method for infectious diseases. The Journal of Infusional Chemotherapy. 2009;**15**(2):62-69

[61] Lin Y-P, Lee D-W, McDonough SP, Nicholson L, Sharma Y, Chang Y-F. The repeated domains of *Leptospira* immunoglobulin-like proteins interact with elastin and tropoealstin. Journal of Biological Chemistry. 2009;**284**(29):19380-19391

[62] Alton GD, Berke O, Reid-Smith R, Ojkic D, Prescott JF. Increase in seroprevalence of canine leptospirosis and its risk factors, Ontario 1998-2006. Canadian Journal of Veterinary Research. 2009;**73**(3):167

[63] Winslow WE, Merry DJ, Pirc ML, Devine PL. Evaluation of a commercial enzyme-linked immunosorbent assay for detection of immunoglobulin M antibody in diagnosis of human leptospiral infection. Journal of Clinical Microbiology. 1997;**35**(8):1938-1942

[64] Braunwald E, Fauci A, Kasper A. Harrison's Principles of Internal Medicine. New York: McGrawHill; 2001

[65] Mcclain JBL, Ballou WR, Harrison SM, Steinweg DL. Doxycycline therapy for leptospirosis. Annals of Internal Medicine. 1984;**100**(5):696-698

[66] Daher EDF, Nogueira CB. Evaluation of penicillin therapy in patients with leptospirosis and acute renal failure. Revista do Instituto de Medicina Tropical de São Paulo. 2000;**42**(6):327-332

[67] Suputtamongkol Y, Niwattayakul K, Suttinont C, Losuwanaluk K, Limpaiboon R, Chierakul W, et al. An open, randomized, controlled trial of penicillin, doxycycline, and cefotaxime for patients with severe leptospirosis. Clinical Infectious Diseases. 2004;**39**(10):1417-1424

[68] Panaphut T, Domrongkitchaiporn S, Vibhagool A, Thinkamrop B, Susaengrat W. Ceftriaxone compared with sodium penicillin G for treatment of severe leptospirosis. Clinical Infectious Diseases. 2003;**36**(12):1507-1513

[69] Niwattayakul K, Kaewtasi S, Chueasuwanchai S, Hoontrakul S, Chareonwat S, Suttinont C, et al. An open randomized controlled trial of desmopressin and pulse dexamethasone as adjunct therapy in patients with pulmonary involvement associated with severe leptospirosis. Clinical Microbiology and Infection. 2010;**16**(8):1207-1212

[70] Karande S, Satam N, Kulkarni M, Bharadwaj R, Pol S. Leptospiral pneumonia. Indian Journal of Pediatrics. 2005;**72**(1):86

[71] Ozkanlar Y, Aktas M, Kaynar O, Ozkanlar S, Celebi F. Efficacy of blood transfusion accompanied by antibiotics and B vitamins for the treatment of naturally occurring leptospirosis in cattle. Revista de Medicina Veterinaria. 2010;**161**(7):336-341

[72] Thompson JC, Manktelow B. Pathogenesis and red blood cell destruction in haemoglobinaemic leptospirosis. Journal of Comparative Pathology. 1986;**96**(5):529-540

[73] Goarant C. Leptospirosis: Risk factors and management challenges in developing countries. Research and Reports in Tropical Medicine. 2016;**2016**(7):29-62

[74] Hunt E, Wood B. Use of blood and blood products. Veterinary Clinics: Food Animal Practice. 1999;**15**(3):641-662

[75] Conference PottWDM. Western Dairy Management Conference; 2003

Section 4

Chronic Bacterial Disease of Cattle

Chapter 5

Diseases Caused by Bacteria in Cattle: Tuberculosis

Joseph K.N. Kuria

Abstract

Tuberculosis is an infectious, chronic or acute, localized or disseminated granulomatous disease that affects all animal species, caused by members of the genus mycobacteria. In cattle, the disease is caused by obligatory pathogenic and opportunistic species of mycobacteria and is transmitted between animals mainly through inhalation. It is a major public health concern and humans are infected chiefly through consumption of raw animal products. The disease is characterized by progressive emaciation, which may be terminally fatal. Pathological lesions comprising of be caseous or calcified granulomas are found mainly in the respiratory tract but animals infected through ingestion develop lesions in the lymph nodes of the head and the mesentery. Lesions may disseminate to involve other internal organs and tissues. Histologically, lesions manifest typical granulomas with a necrotic center surrounded by inflammatory cells and a fibrous capsule. Diagnosis is based on history, clinical signs, antemortem tests, and postmortem examination. Culture, isolation, and identification of the organism are confirmatory tests. The disease is a listed under the OIE Terrestrial Animal Health Code and the main method of control is testing and slaughter of affected animals. The importance of the disease is the zoonosis, loss in productivity in affected animals, and the cost of control.

Keywords: bacterial diseases, cattle, mycobacteria

1. Introduction

Tuberculosis in cattle is of serious public health as well as economic concern worldwide but more so in developing world. The disease is a zoonosis, transmitted from animals to humans mainly through the consumption of raw animal products especially milk. Human infections are therefore prevalent in communities with poor food hygiene and unsanitary cultural practices [1]. The resultant disease manifestation is largely similar to the human-type tuberculosis, with socioeconomic costs of stigma, reduced productivity, mortality, and cost of treatment. Rigorous control and eradication programs have drastically reduced transmission to humans in the developed world but in the developing world, it remains a serious threat to human health. Animal to animal transmission is mainly through the inhalation of infective respiratory aerosols. Production systems that involve close contact between animals promote transmission. The disease is listed under World Animal Health Organization (OIE) and therefore a restriction to trade in animals and animal products. Other costs include reduced animal productivity and the cost of control.

 IntechOpen

Since its identification in 1898, *Mycobacterium bovis* (later split into two subspecies: *M. bovis* subsp. *bovis* and *M. bovis* subsp. *caprae*) has been considered as the etiological agent of tuberculosis but later, other members of the *Mycobacterium tuberculosis* complex (MTBC) were found to cause similar infections [2–4]. More recently, species of mycobacteria hitherto regarded as saprophytic and nonpathogenic, referred to as nontuberculous mycobacteria (NTM) and more recently, mycobacteria other than tuberculosis (MOTTs) have been identified as causative agents [4, 5]. Apart from the requirement for isolation and identification of the causative for confirmatory diagnosis, these species have complicated interpretation of in vivo diagnostic tests, such as the tuberculin test, due to the expected cross-reactive immune responses [6, 7]. Some of these MOTTs have also been found to cause a variety of infections in humans and should therefore be considered potentially as zoonotic, and infestations in cattle and other animals as important and the MTBC. Many other species of animals are also susceptible to *M. bovis*. These include wildlife species, which constitute reservoirs of infection for domestic animals [8, 9]. Transmission to domestic animals and humans is therefore potentially an outcome of human-wildlife conflict. With such a variety of mycobacteria species, now associated with tuberculosis in cattle, perhaps the etiological term mycobacteriosis, rather than the pathological term tuberculosis, should be more applicable. This chapter will explore the etiology, epidemiology, pathogenesis, pathology, diagnosis, public health importance, and control of tuberculosis in cattle. It is expected that the chapter will be found useful by veterinary students, tutors, animal health service providers, and researchers.

2. Definition

Tuberculosis is an infectious, chronic or acute, localized or disseminated granulomatous disease that affects mammals, fish, and birds, caused by members of the genus *Mycobacterium*. In cattle, the disease is caused by obligatory pathogenic and opportunistic species of mycobacteria. Animals affected by the disseminated infection progressively emaciate and finally succumb to the infection. The importance of the disease is its zoonosis and the economic losses it causes.

3. History

Tuberculosis affects warm- and cold-blooded animals and it is estimated that it has been around for more than 3 million years [10]. The disease in cattle was first observed by the Spaniard farmer, Lucius Junius Moderatus Columella in Northern Italy in the year 14 AD [11]. In 1881, Robert Koch discovered *Mycobacterium tuberculosis* (tubercle bacillus) as the cause of tuberculosis in humans and in 1882, established the connection between human and animal tuberculosis through the observation that consumption of contaminated cow's milk led to infection. In 1898, Theobald Smith identified *M. bovis* as a different species from *M. tuberculosis*. The first compulsory milk pasteurization law was enacted in UK in 1908 following the research that linked consumption of raw milk to extrapulmonary tuberculosis; two French scientists Albert Calmette and Camille Guerin developed the Bacillus Calmette-Guerin (BCG) vaccine for immunizing humans against tuberculosis, by attenuating *M. bovis* through subculture. The vaccine was first used in 1921 [12]. In 1890, Robert Koch extracted tuberculin from the tubercle bacilli. The extract was initially tried as a vaccine, but later shown to have diagnostic potential to detect infected animals. The tuberculin skin test for animals was thereafter developed [10]. The development of the skin test for humans was then carried out by Von Pirquet and Mantoux in 1907–1908 [13]. In the developed world, bovine TB eradication programs involving herd testing and culling of reactors and pasteurization of milk has largely eliminated the spread of bovine TB. The disease, however, remains a serious public health problem in many developing countries [14].

4. Etiology

4.1 Classification of mycobacteria

The genus *Mycobacterium* is the only genus in the family *Mycobacteraceae* in the order *Actinomycetales*, which includes other mycolic acid-containing genera, namely *Nocadia*, *Rhodococcus*, *Gordonia*, and *Tsukamurlla*. Currently, the genus comprises of over 150 species and 13 subspecies [15, 16]. Within the genus, classification is based on several factors including growth rate and pathogenicity. Based on pathogenicity, it can be classified into two groups: tuberculous and nontuberculous mycobacteria, the latter also referred to as mycobacteria other than tuberculosis (MOTTs). A refined classification on this basis groups the genus into obligatory pathogens, potentially pathogenic (opportunistic) and saprophytic or ubiquitous microorganisms [17]. Obligatory pathogens belong to *Mycobacterium tuberculosis* complex (MTBC) group that comprise *Mycobacterium bovis* subsp. *bovis, M. bovis* subsp. *caprae, M. tuberculosis, M. africanum, M. bovis BCG, M. canetti, M. microtti, M. pinnipedii,* and *M. leprae* [18]. All MTBC species have identical 16S rRNA sequences and a 99.9% similarity at nucleotide level, and may even be considered subspecies, but differ significantly in their host range [19]. The potentially pathogenic mycobacteria, represented by the *Mycobacterium avium* complex (MAC), consists of closely related species and subspecies, which include, among others, *M. avium* subsp. *avium, M. avium* subsp. *paratuberculosis*, and *M. avium* subsp. *hominissuis*. The potentially pathogenic species are found in the environment as well as in the susceptible hosts and cause disease mainly in hosts with compromised immunity [20]. Saprophytic mycobacteria are the largest group found in the environment. Some, such as *M. kansasii, M. asiaticum, M. interjectum, M. szulgai, M. fortuitum, M. celatum, M. ulcerans, M. smegmatis*, and *M. septicum* have been associated with diseases in humans and animals [21].

On the basis of growth rate, the genus is classified into slow and rapidly growing species, with rapid-growers being those that produce grossly visible colonies in less than 7 days and slow-growers taking over 7 days. Slow-growing species are more commonly associated with pathogenicity than the fast-growing group [22].

In cattle and other ruminants, tuberculosis is caused mainly by the obligate pathogen *Mycobacterium bovis* subsp. *bovis* but infections by *Mycobacterium bovis* subsp. *caprae*, *Mycobacterium tuberculosis* and *Mycobacterium africanum* also occur [2–4]. In Central Europe, *M. bovis* subsp. *capra*e is the major cause of tuberculosis in cattle [23, 24]. The disease caused by *M. bovis* subsp. *bovis and M. bovis* subsp. *caprae* is commonly referred to as bovine or zoonotic tuberculosis. Although not as widely as zoonotic tuberculosis, MOTTs infections have been reported in cattle exhibiting granulomatous lesions identical to those caused by the MTBC complex [6, 15, 16].

4.2 Cellular morphology and staining

Mycobacteria are nonmotile, noncapsulating, and nonspore forming rods measuring 0.2–0.6 µm by 1.0–10 µm with a slender, straight or slightly curved shape. The cell wall of mycobacteria contains a hydrophobic lipid layer, which includes mycolic acids, phosphatidylinositol, mannosides, phthiocerol dimycocerosates, isoprenoid lipids, glycerophospholipids, lipoarabinomannan, and trehalose mycolates and lipoglycans, which give the organism some unique characteristics:

1. Growth requires complex organic media, containing long-chain free fatty acids necessary for the synthesis of the lipid layer.

2. The hydrophobic lipid layer causes poor penetration of nutrients, hence the slow growth of the organism and the long incubation period of disease.

3. The poor penetration of chemical agents makes the organism difficult to stain by ordinary procedures. Once stained, they resist decolorization even by weak mineral acids such as 3% hydrochloric acid in ethanol, hence the name acid-fast bacilli (AFB). Mycobacteria have a cell wall structure characteristic of Gram-positive bacteria but they cannot be stained by this method although they may stain weakly Gram-positive.

4. The organism is highly resistant to disinfectants and most antibiotics, occasioning lengthy treatment of infection.

5. The presence of fatty acids in the cell wall causes cells to aggregate in a pattern referred to as "cording," observed in stained smears and in broth cultures, due to resemblance to strands of rope cords, and in solid media, growth resembles that of fungi (*myco* = Greek = means "fungus").

6. The lipid layer plays a role in resistance to the host's immune system [25–27]. Paradoxically, the biosynthesis site of some of the lipid components is also the site of action of anti-TB drugs [26].

4.3 Cultural characteristics

Mycobacteria are obligate aerobes and require complex organic media for growth. Solid media such as the egg-based Lowenstein-Jensen, (L-J), Middlebrook 7H10, and Middlebrook 7H11 or liquid media such as Modified Middlebrook 7H9 broth are used. Like other MTBC members, *M. bovis* is a slow grower. On solid media, colonies are detectable 3–6 and up to 12 weeks of incubation at 37°C weeks depending on the concentration of inoculum [28]. Colonies are small, raised, rounded, off-white (bluff) in color, wrinkled surface, and with irregular margins [29]. Addition of pyruvate is reported to stimulate growth of *M. bovis* and glycerol, which favors growth of *M. tuberculosis,* is said to inhibit it [28, 30]. Other findings however, indicate that *M. bovis* can grow satisfactorily in media containing either substance [5]. Members of MTBC group, including *M. bovis,* are inhibited by paranitrobenzoic acid (PNB), a criteria used to differentiate the group from MOTTs [31, 32]. Growth in liquid media is faster since the organism is surrounded by the media and access to nutrients is more efficient. Growth appears as clumps or "cords." Addition of egg yolk to the growth medium enhances growth, due to the presence of phospholipids that are required for growth but synthetic phospholipids such as polyoxyethylene sorbate compounds (Tweens) can also be used, which also lower the tendency of the mycobacteria to aggregate, giving a diffuse homogenous turbidity [33].

4.4 Biochemical properties

M. bovis exhibits strain variation in biochemical characteristics, which can be summarized as follows [28, 34, 35]:

Test	Reaction	
	M. bovis	*M. tuberculosis*
Sensitivity to thiophen-2-carboxylic acid hydrazide (TCH)	+	—
Sensitivity isonicotinic acid hydrazide (INH)	+	+
Niacin production	—	+
Nitrate reduction	—	+
Pyrazinamidase test	+*	—
Nicotinamidase test	+*	—
Amidase test	—	+
Urease production	+	Variable
Growth under microaerophilic environment	+	—

*Mycobacterium bovis *subsp.* caprae *is negative.*

The main limitation of biochemical tests is that sufficient amounts of bacterial cells as well and several weeks of incubation are required. The other limitation is that unknown species of mycobacteria cannot be identified. The availability of more rapid methods such as molecular methods has therefore diminished the use of biochemical tests.

4.5 Environmental, chemical, and drug resistance

In general, mycobacteria are inactivated by prolonged exposure to heat, direct sunlight, and dry conditions. They are killed by temperatures of 65°C and above for at least 30 minutes and UV light but are resistant to freezing for prolonged periods. Under ordinary temperatures, *M. bovis* can persist in slurry and soil for at least 6 months and can survive for long periods in buildings and transport vehicles under dark, cold, and moist conditions [29, 36, 37]. The high lipid and wax content makes mycobacteria less susceptible to many chemical agents and disinfectants. Chemicals such as quaternary ammonium compounds, hexachlorophene, and chlorhexidine have bacteriostatic effect while formaldehyde vapor, chlorine compounds, 70% ethanol, hydrogen peroxide alkaline glutaraldehyde, and 5% phenol have bactericidal effect. Although treatment of infected animals is not normally practiced, *M. bovis* is resistant to most antibiotics but sensitive to the drugs used in treatment of *M. tuberculosis* (rifampin, isoniazid, streptomycin (STR), and ethambutol). *M. bovis* subsp. *bovis* is resistant to pyrazinamide (PZA), a first-line TB treatment drug in humans [38]. This characteristic is relevant in the management of infection in humans and also useful in differentiating *M. bovis* from *M. tuberculosis*. Multi-drug resistant strains of *M. bovis* have been reported in many countries [39].

5. Epidemiology of bovine tuberculosis

5.1 Host range

Mycobacteria have one of the widest host range and affects mammal, birds, fish, reptiles, and amphibians. Cattle and related ruminants such as buffalo and bison are regarded as the main hosts of *M. bovis* subspecies. Other mammalian hosts include sheep, goats, camels, horses, llamas, pigs, dogs, cats, humans, and nonhuman primates [40]. Many wild animals, including elephants, rhinoceroses, coyotes, mink, otters, seals, sea lions, hares, bears, warthogs, large cats ferrets, and rodents are affected. Known maintenance hosts include possums and ferrets in New Zealand; badgers, raccoons, and foxes in Europe; bison and elk in Canada; and kudu and African buffalo in Africa and white-tailed deer in the USA [9].

5.2 Geographical distribution and prevalence

Zoonotic tuberculosis caused by *M. bovis* has a worldwide distribution. It was reported by 78 of the 181 OIE reporting countries in 2017, distributed in every region of the world [41]. This figure is likely to be much lower due to under-reporting, occasioned by inadequate surveillance. Globally, the prevalence has been estimated at 0.8% [42]. Using reports of zoonotic tuberculosis in humans as indication, the highest prevalence is found in African region followed by South East Asia, Western pacific, Eastern Mediterranean, Europe, and lastly Americas [43]. The disease has been largely controlled in developed world through systematic test and slaughter of infected animals, meat inspection surveillance in abattoirs, and milk pasteurization but complete eradication has been hindered by the existence of reservoirs of the agent in wildlife species [44]. In many developing countries, the disease remains largely neglected [45]. MOTTs have mainly been isolated coincidentally from animal lesions while searching for *M. bovis*. Isolation of MOOTs from cattle carcasses range approximately between 7 and 70% of total isolates [4, 5].

5.3 Transmission and risk factors

Infected animals shed *Mycobacterium* via respiratory aerosols, milk, saliva, feces, urine, and discharging lesions. The main route of infection in cattle is mainly through the inhalation of infective aerosols. This is supported by high frequency of tuberculous lesions found in the respiratory tract and associated lymph nodes [46]. Transmission is facilitated by close contact between animals and therefore the production system plays an important role. Intensive livestock farming, referred to as zero-grazing, promotes close contact between animals. In extensive production, such as practiced by nomadic pastoralists in arid and semiarid regions of Africa, close contact between animals occur in, night shelters, watering points, vaccination centers, marketing yards, and at dipping tanks while in intensive production close contact occurs during milking and in watering and feeding troughs [36]. Ingestion of contaminated feed and water is generally considered to be a secondary, less important route of transmission but in countries where untreated manure is commonly used as a fertilizer in farms, such manure can become a source of infection to animals through pasture and vegetation contamination [36, 37]. The oral route is also particularly important in calves nursing from infected cows.

Other rare routes of infection include cutaneous, genital during coitus, congenital through placental or umbilical infection, and transmission through udder infections [47]. Contact between domestic and wild animals through pasture contamination is a risk factor. Domestic species reported to be reservoirs and spill-over hosts include sheep and goats. The low prevalence of tuberculosis in these species in the African region, however, indicates that they may not be significant in transmission of disease to cattle [48, 49].

Human to animal transmission through aerosols is well documented and patients with pulmonary tuberculosis pose danger to animals [50]. Humans with urogenital tuberculosis represent a source of infection for animals through contamination of pastures with urine. In Ethiopia, the traditional practice of spiting chewed tobacco into mouths of livestock as anti-parasitic treatment is a potential source of infection with *M. tuberculosis* [3].

Male animals were more significantly affected by than female animals while *Bos indicus* (zebu) have been found to be more resistant than *Bos Taurus* (Exotic breeds). At the herd level, herd size increases infection due to increased exposure and introduction of new animals into a herd is a risk factor [51].

The primary source of infection by MOTTs is presumably the environment [16], and although, the specific source of individual infections may not be easily identified, and the route of infection may be deduced from the localization of granulomas.

6. Pathogenesis

Animals exposed by ingestion of contaminated feed or water often develop primary foci in lymph nodes associated with the intestinal tract, while aerosol exposure leads to the involvement of the lungs and associated lymph nodes. In case of respiratory infection, the mucociliary clearance in the upper respiratory passages may prevent infection in some exposed animals [52]. In the bronchi, the organism penetrates the mucosa and are trapped and phagocytosed in the bronchial and mediastinal lymph nodes. In the lungs, the bacterial are phagocytosed by alveolar macrophages. In case of oral infection, the organism presumably penetrates the bucal or intestinal mucosa and, via the lymphatics, reaches the phagocytes in the draining lymph node. The phagocytosis causes a localized inflammatory reaction and recruitment of mononuclear cells from neighboring blood vessels. The cellular response results in the accumulation of large number of phagocytes leading to the formation of the granuloma or the tubercle that characterizes the disease [36, 47]. The granuloma consists of infected macrophages surrounded by epithelioid cells, granulocytes, lymphocytes, and later, multinucleated giant cells [53].

Mycobacteria are facultative intracellular pathogens, and survive and multiply within the hosts' phagocyte. The ability of the organism to survive intracellular within macrophages involves interfering with the development of the phagosome into a degradative vesicle. It is thought that the organism prevents the phagosome from maturing and fusing with lysosomes to form the phagolysosome. The mycolic acids of the organism are thought to play a role in blocking this phagosome maturation [54, 55]. Some components of the lipid layer, such trehalose dimycolate, may cause death of macrophages by direct cytotoxicity [52]. The *Mycobacterium* survival and multiplication within the phagosomes eventually destroys the macrophage. When entering into the death phase, infected macrophages release mycobacterial antigens, which are engulfed by uninfected dendritic cells, processed and subsequently presented, via major histocompatibility complex class I, to CD8+ T cells. The cellular hypersensitivity that develops, contributes to cell death and tissue destruction resulting in caseous necrosis. In some instances, liquefaction and cavity formation occur as a result of enzymatic action on proteins and lipids, and the organism multiplies uncontrolled in these cavities. Rapture of the cavities into the bronchi allows aerosol spread of the bacilli. Dissemination by bacteria-containing macrophage may occur through vascular and lymphatic channels to form lesions in many organs, as in acute miliary TB, which is rapidly fatal [47, 53]. Innate non-specific and specific cell-mediated immunities are the main host defense mechanisms. The innate resistance may clear the initial infection and prevent mycobacteria to proliferate. Specific resistance is mediated by T-lymphocytes. They destroy infected macrophages or activate them to destroy extracellular bacilli through soluble mediators such as gamma interferon [56]. Where the host has been able to contain spread of infection, lesions consistency progress from caseous, fibro-caseous, fibro-calcified to calcified and are surrounded by a fibrous capsule. Calcified granulomas generally indicate a successful suppression of the infection by the immune response and the lesions may regress completely [53]. During pathological processes, mycobacteria are present in tuberculous tissue and in various body fluids, secretions and excretions such as milk, blood, sputum, bronchoalveolar lavages, cerebrospinal fluid, and semen [36].

7. Pathology

Pathology of tuberculosis is characterized by the formation of granulomatous lesions mainly in the respiratory and alimentary tracts and associated lymph nodes.

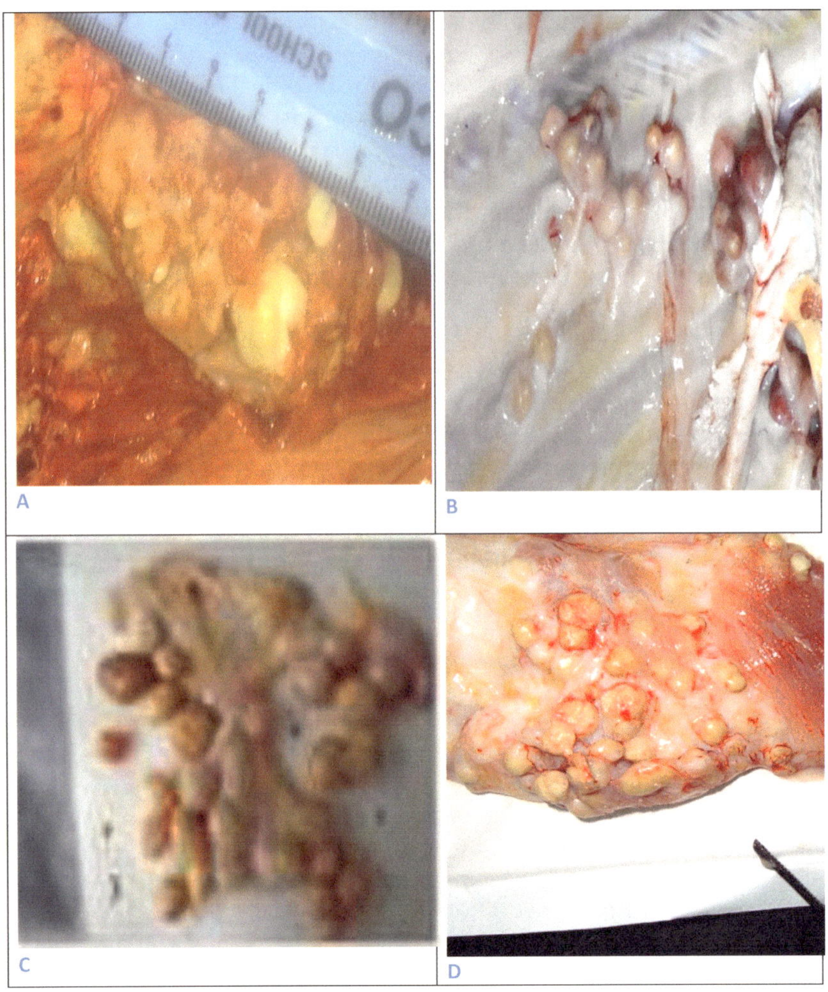

Figure 1.
Multiple tuberculosis lesions observed in lungs (A), pleura (B), mesentery (C) and diaphragm (D) in cattle during postmortem meat inspection.

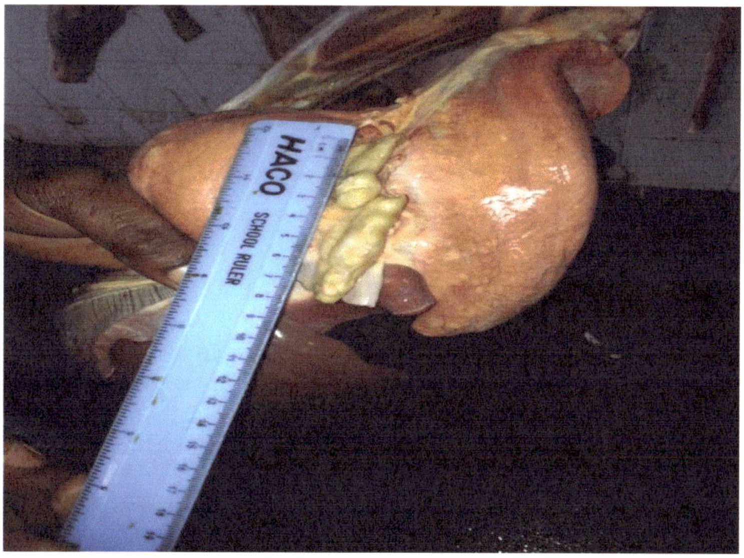

Figure 2.
Tuberculous lesions in the mediastinal lymph nodes of a goat meat carcass. ©2018. JKN Kuria.

The lesions may be localized to few organs or tissues or disseminated to multiple sites. In the respiratory system, lesions are observed in bronchial lymph nodes, in lungs (**Figure 1A**) and in mediastinal lymph nodes (**Figure 2**). The alimentary system lesions involve the retropharyngeal, parotid, sub-maxillary, and mesenteric lymph nodes (**Figure 1C**), as well as the liver and portal lymph nodes, the spleen and other internal organs such as the kidneys [28]. Lesions may also be found on surfaces of body cavities such as the pleura (**Figure 1B**), diaphragm (**Figure 1D**), and peritoneum. In most cases, lesions are confined to the lymph nodes of the head region and respiratory tract [47]. The size, color, and consistency of the lesions vary widely according to the stage of infection. Lesion sizes are microscopic or large enough to involve the greater part of or the whole organ or tissue. The consistency ranges from caseopurulent, fibro-caseous fibro-calcified to calcified, but may also be thin-walled purulent cavities [4, 5, 53]. Histopathological features of a granuloma show a central area of caseous necrosis with or without calcification, surrounded by macrophages, lymphocytes, plasma cells, neutrophils, epithelioid cells, and Langhan's giant cells and enclosed partially or completely by a fibrous capsule [53].

8. Clinical signs

The signs of tuberculosis in cattle usually vary depending on the organ systems affected. In the early stages, clinical signs are not visible and many animals with tuberculosis are clinically normal. The signs have a gradual onset characterized by progressive weakness, debility, and mild fluctuating fever. Advanced lung involvement is characterized by dyspnea, chronic moist cough, more marked in the morning and during cold weather, and reduced exercise tolerance [14]. Swollen lymph nodes of the head may be observed and involvement of internal lymph nodes may result in obstruction signs of the system or organ affected. There may be diarrhea or constipation due gastrointestinal tract involvement. Mammary tuberculosis has been found in varying proportions of animals, from 1 to 2%, up to 5.4% and is characterized by persistent mastitis and hypertrophy [40]. Infertility or abortion may result from tuberculous metritis, accompanied by chronic purulent vaginal discharge. Affected animals generally remain bright and alert and maintain a good appetite despite weakness and sluggishness [57]. Acute or subacute death may result from military tuberculosis, caused by rapid widespread dissemination, from primary or secondary lesions through the hematogenous route.

9. Public health importance

Zoonotic tuberculosis in cattle is a public health concern worldwide. The prevalence is estimated at 0.5–1% in developed countries and 10–15% in developing countries [58]. In developing world, high levels of human immunodeficiency virus (HIV) and poverty, especially in Sub-Saharan countries, are contributing factors. Consumption of raw or undercooked products, and especially milk, from infected cattle is the main cause of nonpulmonary tuberculosis [59]. *M. bovis* is excreted in milk of about 1–2% of infected cattle in large numbers such that a single infected cow can contaminate bulk milk by 100 cows to cause infection in susceptible humans [60]. Social-cultural factors, for instance, the tradition by pastoral communities to consume raw blood and milk and raw or undercooked meat and meat products, are risk factors [1]. It is estimated that in Africa, 90% of milk is consumed either raw or fermented, thus increasing the risk of transmission [61]. Cervical lymphadenitis is the commonest manifestation of oral infection (**Figure 3**). Inhalation of infected dust particles or aerosols shed by infected cattle is the second important route especially in rural pastoralist communities. Abattoir workers, farmers, milkers, veterinarians, and animal handlers are also exposed to this mode of transmission [58, 62]. Infection in wildlife puts hunters, trappers, and zoo workers at risk. Trans-cutaneous transmission may occur through handling of infected carcasses [47].

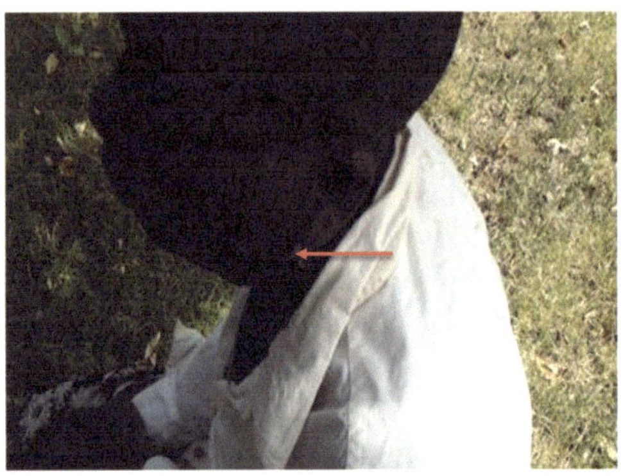

Figure 3.
Raptured lesion (arrowed) in the left retropharyngeal lymph node of a tuberculosis patient infected by M. bovis. *©2018 JKN Kuria.*

10. Diagnosis

Tuberculosis in cattle can be diagnosed in live animals and also during postmortem examination of dead or slaughtered carcasses. In live animals, clinical signs, tuberculin skin test, and gamma interferon assay can be used. At postmortem, pathological lesions and acid fast staining are preliminary tests while culture and DNA analysis are confirmatory.

10.1 Diagnosis by clinical signs

Clinical diagnosis may be difficult due to the chronic nature of the disease and the wide variety of symptoms, resembling other chronic debilitating conditions. The disease should be suspected on the basis of history coupled with signs of progressive emaciation, in spite of good appetite, fluctuating temperature, chronic, and moist cough dysphagia and noisy breathing. Enlargement of supramammary lymph nodes may be observed. Differential diagnosis includes contagious bovine pleuropneumonia, pasteurellosis *Trueperella pyogenes* pneumonia, bovine lymphosarcoma, traumatic pericarditis, and fascioliasis [63]. Animals suspected of tuberculosis infection should be thoroughly examined by palpation of all superficial lymph nodes, the udder in females and percussion and auscultation of the pulmonary area.

10.2 Tuberculin skin test

Tuberculin skin test is the standard procedure recommended by the World Organization for Animal Health (OIE) for the diagnosis of bovine TB in live animals. This test measures the delayed type hypersensitivity response to tuberculin, *referred* to as purified protein derivative (PPD), injected intradermally. There are two variations of the test. The single intradermal test (SITT), which uses PPD from *M. bovis* only (PPD-B), and the comparative intradermal test (CITT), which uses PPD-B and PPD from *Mycobacteria avium*, (PPD-A). In the SITT, PPD-B is injected intradermally in the neck region. A positive test is indicated by a delayed hypersensitivity reaction (**Figure 4**). The skin thickness at injection site is measured with a pair of calipers before and 72 hours after injection. A relative change greater than 4 mm in skin thickness at the site is considered positive for *M. bovis* infection [28]. The CITT is designed to address the cross-reaction between *M. bovis* and the *M. avium*. PPD-B and PPD-A are injected side by side, around 12 cm apart, and skin swelling is measured after 72 hours. The test result is considered positive, if the relative difference in the increase of skin thickness at the site of PPD-B injection is 4 mm greater than that at the site of PPD-A injection [28]. The sensitivity and specificity of the CITT has been estimated at 81–85 and 80.0, and 99.9%,

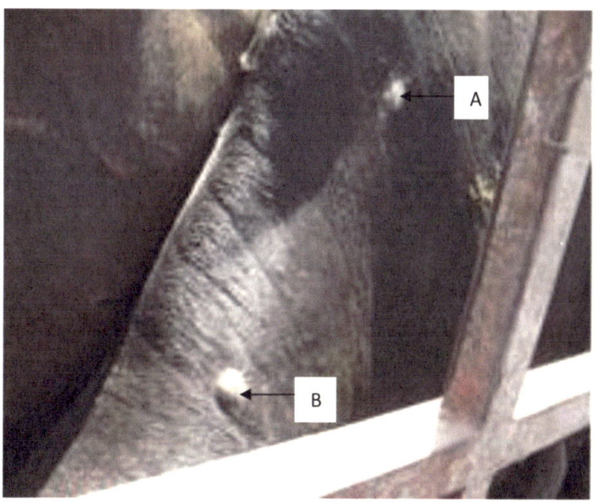

Figure 4.
A comparative intradermal tuberculin test in a cow showing a positive reaction. PPD-A was injected at site A and PPD-B at site B. ©2018. JKN Kuria.

respectively [58, 64]. The CTT has higher specificity than the SITT since it can distinguish animals infected with nontuberculous mycobacteria, specifically the MAC complex, which include *M. avium* subsp. *paratuberculosis*, the causative agent of Johne's disease. Other MOTTs species with ability to cross-react with *M. bovis* have, however, been isolated from tuberculous lesion in cattle and related wild species. The advantage of the CITT over the SITT is therefore limited [5–7].

10.3 Gamma interferon assays

The gamma interferon assay (IFN*γ)* is an *in vitro* form of the CITT. It is based on detection of *γ* interferon produced by specific circulating lymphocytes upon stimulation of heparinized whole blood *in vitro* with PPD-B and PPD-A. Detection of IFN*γ* is carried by a sandwich ELISA, using two monoclonal antibodies to bovine gamma-interferon, after incubation of the blood for about 16–24 hours with PPD-B and PPD-A. The IFN*γ* test is reportedly more sensitive than the tuberculin test and can detect infected animals that are negative to the later. The sensitivity and specificity are estimated at 81.8 and 99.1% [65]. It has been observed that more infected cattle can be identified by using both the tuberculin and the IFN*γ* tests and it is recommended that both tests be conducted in parallel [66]. The advantage of the IFNγ is that infected animals are detected early and only one visit to the farm is required. It is particularly convenient for animals that are difficult to capture or handle, such as cattle reared in ranches or under nomadic pastoralism, or wildlife, as they need only to be captured once rather than twice. It however requires more technical expertise and facilities and is costly (approximately 10 USD, for consumable materials per test).

10.4 Postmortem diagnosis

Detection of tuberculosis using pathological examination involves visual observation, palpation, and incision of organs and tissue to detect lesions. A presumptive diagnosis can be made on the basis of macroscopic granulomatous lesions (**Figures 1** and **2**). Differential diagnosis includes parasitic and mycotic granulomas and abscesses caused by other bacterial pathogens such as *Actinomyces bovis*, *Actinobacillosis,* and *Trueperella pyogenes*, as well as bovine lymphosarcoma [67, 68]. Further, very small lesions may be missed and may only be detected microscopically. Routine postmortem meat inspection has been found to detect approximately only 47% of presumptive lesions [69]. Direct smears of suspected lesions should be stained by the acid fast method and examined for acid-fast bacilli (**Figure 5**).

10.5 Culture and isolation of mycobacteria

Culture is considered the "gold standard" for detection of *Mycobacteria* [69]. Samples for culture are first homogenized and decontaminated with sodium hydroxide to inactivate any contaminant bacteria present in the sample, inoculated into solid or liquid media and incubated at 37°C. Solid media include egg-based Lowenstein-Jensen (L-J), Agar-based media such as Middlebrook 7H10, 7H11, and Stonebrink Leslie solid culture media. Solid media is prepared as slants in screw-capped bottles. In Lowenstein-Jensen media, malachite green dye (0.025 g/100 ml) is used as a selective agent. Isolation should target MTBC and MOTTs and it is recommended that each sample is inoculated into three tubes of LJ, one containing glycerol, another pyruvate, and the other PNB. Most mycobacteria are obligatory aerobic but *M. bovis* is microaerophilic. Screw caps should be loosened, to allow in oxygen, and the tubes incubated in a slanting position, to allow bacteria to seed onto

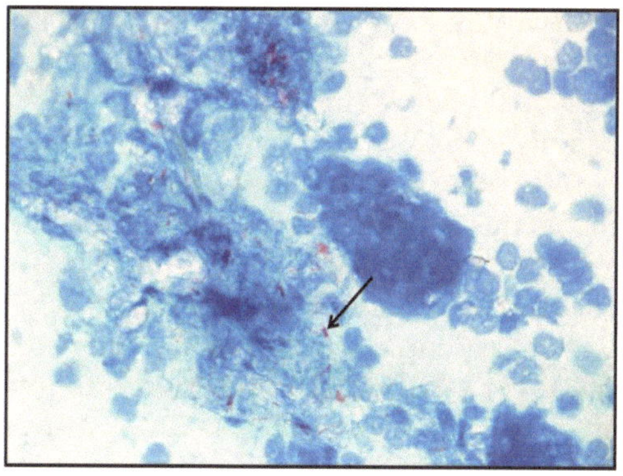

Figure 5.
Direct smear of a tuberculous lymph node lesion from a cow, showing presence of acid-fast bacilli (arrowed). ZN × 1000. ©2018. JKN Kuria.

the media. Thereafter, the caps are tightened and the tubes incubated vertically for six 12 weeks. Liquid media include BACTEC 460, Mycobacterial Growth Indicator Tube (MGIT), which have enriched Middlebrook 7Ha with antibiotics and growth promoters are added. BACTEC 460 MGIT media is fully automated and can monitor the growth of mycobacteria by the use of oxygen quenching or fluorescent sensor. Mycobacteria may not be recovered in the cultures for a number of reasons:

1. Extended period between sample collection and analysis, leading to death of the organism.

2. Nonviability of the bacilli due to necrosis and calcification of granulomas.

3. Organisms may be inactivated by the decontamination process.

4. Samples may contain microorganisms other than mycobacteria.

Cultures suspected to be mycobacteria are then stained by acid fast method for confirmation. All laboratory procedures must be conducted in a class II biosafety cabinet in a laboratory environment that has been found safe and secure following risk assessment.

10.6 Molecular diagnosis

Molecular tools for differentiating *Mycobacterium* species have been developed [70]. Polymerase chain reaction (PCR) technique involves detection of the genetic material that is unique and specific to a species. Convenient commercial kits are available. Genotype *Mycobacterium* (Hain, Nehren, and Germany) are line probe assays available in three different formats: Genotype MTBC differentiate species in MTBC; GenoType *Mycobacterium* common mycobacteria (CM) detects most frequently encountered Mycobacteria species and Genotype *Mycobacterium* additional species (AS) detects less frequently encountered Mycobacteria species. This kit uses reverse hybridization technology on a solid membrane matrix consisting of nitrocellulose strips. The DNA probes are immobilized on parallel lines on the strips. Biotinylated DNA apricon fragments of the 16S-23SrRNA spacer region are incubated with the labeled strips and hybridization detected colorimetrically by addition of an enzyme, Streptavidin-alkaline phosphatase, and a chromogenic substrate. A precipitate is formed on the membrane, where hybridization takes place. Another line probe assay is INNOLiPa Mycobacteria (Innogenetics, Ghent, Belgium). Line probe assays are convenient in that they can detect many species of mycobacteria simultaneously. The strips can also be conveniently dried and preserved.

AccuProbe (GEN-Probe, San Diego, California, USA), is an in-solution hybridization assay. DNA probes consisting of species-specific, single-stranded DNA oligonucleotides are prepared complementary to ribosomal RNA released from bacterial cultures and labeled with acridinum ester (chemiluminescent). Hybridization is measured by chemiluminescence using a luminometer and expressed as relative light units (RLU). The test can be performed on culture growing from broth or solid media and will detect all members of MTBC but without differentiating the species. However, since no nucleic acid amplification occurs in the assay, identification requires sufficient growth.

Real-time commercial PCR kits are also available for direct detection in clinical specimens and pathological specimens but can also be used for identification of cultures. The current available kits detect MTBC but not individual species.

Restriction fragment length polymorphism (RFLP) or spoligotyping distinguishes between phenotypically different strains of *M. bovis* [71]. It is designed to detect the unique spacers within the direct repeat (DR) locus of the *M. bovis* genome [72] and is a useful epidemiological tool, in that it indicates strains circulating in a population, and therefore the transmission patterns.

DNA tests are more rapid and reliable than the conventional identification methods, but are still limited to the postmortem diagnosis of the infection, in that, tissue samples or isolates are still required. Extraction and detection DNA in nasal swab samples, milk, lymph node aspirates may however be achieved [73].

11. Economic impact

Economic losses due to tuberculosis in cattle worldwide are estimated at more than US $3 billion annually [74]. This may be an underestimate since losses in many developing countries have not been examined sufficiently or studied at all. Loss of productivity of infected animals includes reduced milk yields, meat production, and reduced fertility. Among dairy cattle, milk production may decrease between 4 and 18%. Other direct losses include mortalities, infertility, calf mortalities, additional processing for infected animals, and condemnation of carcasses at slaughterhouses. Export market restrictions constitute nontariff barriers to trade. The cost of control involves meat inspection, test and slaughter of positive animals, pasteurization of milk, and compensation schemes to farmers. The public health cost include cost of treatment, mortality, loss of incomes and livelihoods, food insecurity, stigmatization as well as extra working hours for those attending to sick humans [75, 76]. Globally, 147,000 new cases of zoonotic TB in humans were estimated in 2016, resulting in 12,500 deaths. Most of the cases were in the African followed by the South-East Asian region [43].

12. Control

Bovine tuberculosis is listed under the OIE Terrestrial Animal Health Code. Control should be aimed at reducing prevalence in animals in order to prevent transmission to humans. The recommended control method in livestock is continuous detection and slaughter of infected animals [28]. Postmortem meat inspection and pasteurization of milk is an effective method of preventing infected animal products from entering the food chain. Meat inspection can allow trace-back to the herd of origin, which can then be tested and eliminated. Individual testing of cattle and removal of infected and in-contact animals, coupled with animal movement controls reduces prevalence [28]. Testing and slaughter may, however, not be tenable in poor countries because of insufficient financial resources, pastoral production method that is characterized by uncontrolled movement of animals, weak veterinary institutions and political instability [28]. Further, in developing countries especially in Africa, cattle are raised together with sheep and goats, which act as reservoirs and are not targets for test and slaughter.

Author details

Joseph K.N. Kuria
Department of Veterinary Pathology, Microbiology and Parasitology, Faculty of Veterinary Medicine, University of Nairobi, Nairobi, Kenya

*Address all correspondence to: jknkuria@uonbi.ac.ke

IntechOpen

© 2019 The Author(s). Licensee IntechOpen. This chapter is distributed under the terms of the Creative Commons Attribution License (http://creativecommons.org/licenses/by/3.0), which permits unrestricted use, distribution, and reproduction in any medium, provided the original work is properly cited.

References

[1] Ameni G, Amenu K, Tibbo M. Bovine tuberculosis: Prevalence and risk factor assessment in cattle and cattle owners in Wuchale-Jida District, Central Ethiopia. Journal of Applied Research in Veterinary Medicine. 2003;**1**:17-26

[2] de Jong BC, Antonio M, Sebastien Gagneux G. *Mycobacterium africanum*—Review of an important cause of human tuberculosis in West Africa. PLoS Neglected Tropical Diseases. 2010;**4**(9): e744. https://doi.org/10.1371/journal.pntd

[3] Ameni G, Martin Vordermeier M, Rebuma Firdessa R, Abraham Aseffa A, Glyn Hewinson G, Gordon SV, et al. *Mycobacterium tuberculosis* infection in grazing cattle in Central Ethiopia. Veterinary Journal. 2011;**188**:359-361. DOI: 10.1016/j.tvjl.2010.05.005. PMCID: PMC3103825. PMID: 20965132

[4] Gathogo SM, Kuria JKN, Ombui JN. Prevalence of bovine tuberculosis in slaughter cattle in Kenya: A postmortem, microbiological and DNA molecular study. Tropical Animal Health and Production. 2012;**44**: 1739-1744. DOI: 10.1007/s11250-012-0131-3

[5] Kuria JKN, Akwalu SK, Muema LM. The etiology and public health significance of mycobacteriosis of cattle in Kenya. International Journal of Mycobacteriology. 2018;7:251-256

[6] Thacker TC, Robbe-Austerman S, Harris B, Palmer MV, Waters WR. Isolation of mycobacteria from clinical samples collected in the United States from 2004 to 2011. BMC Veterinary Research. 2013;**9**:100. DOI: 10.1186/1746-6148-9-100

[7] Gcebe N, Hlokwe TM. Non-tuberculous mycobacteria in south African wildlife: Neglected pathogens and potential impediments for bovine tuberculosis diagnosis. Frontiers in Cellular and Infection Microbiology. 2017;7:15. DOI: 10.3389/fcimb.2017.00015. PMCID: PMC5276850. PMID: 28194371

[8] Aranaz A, De Juan L, Montero N, Sánchez C, Galka M, Delso C, et al. Bovine tuberculosis (*Mycobacterium bovis*) in wildlife in Spain. Journal of Clinical Microbiology. 2004;**42**: 2602-2608. DOI: 10.1128/JCM.42.6.2602-2608.200

[9] Childs JE, Mackenzie JS, Richt JA, editors. Wildlife and Emerging Zoonotic Diseases: The Biology, Circumstances and Consequences of Cross-Species Transmission. Germany: Springer-Verlag, Berlin and Heidelberg; 2007. ISBN 978-3-540-70961-9

[10] Good M, Bakker D, Duignan A, Collins DM. The history of in vivo tuberculin testing in bovine tuberculosis, a "one health" issue. Frontiers in Veterinary Science. 2018;**5**: 59. DOI: 10.3389/fvets.2018.00059

[11] Anonymous. Bobivine TB Essays. 2018. Available from: https://www.megaessays.com/viewpaper/48444.html. [Accessed: September 18, 2018]

[12] Anonymous. History of BCG Vaccine—Calmette, Guerin, Lubeck. 2018. Available from: https://www.tbfacts.org/bcg/. [Accessed: September 18, 2018]

[13] Centre for Disease Control (CDC). Historical Perspectives Centennial: Koch's Discovery of the Tubercle Bacillus. 1982. Available from: https://www.cdc.gov/mmwr/preview/mmwrhtml/00000222.htm

[14] World Organization for Animal Health (OIE). Bovine Tuberculosis.

2018. Available from: http://www.oie.int/fileadmin/Home/eng/Media_Center/docs/pdf/Disease_cards/BOVINE-TB-EN.pdf [Accessed: September 18, 2018]

[15] Gcebe N. The Occurrence and Molecular Characterization of Non-tuberculous Mycobacteria in Cattle, African Buffalo (syncerus caffer) and Their Environments in South Africa and Genomic Characterization and Proteomic Comparison with *Mycobacterium bovis* [PhD thesis]. University of Pretoria; 2015

[16] King HC, Khera-Butler T, Phillip James P, Oakley BB, Erenso G, Aseffa A, et al. Environmental reservoirs of pathogenic mycobacteria across the Ethiopian biogeographical landscape. PLoS One. 2017;**12**(3):e0173811. DOI: 10.1371/journal.pone.0173811

[17] Stanford J, Stanford C. Mycobacteria and their world. International Journal of Mycobacteriology. 2012;**1**:3-12. DOI: 10.1016/j.ijmyco.2012.01.001

[18] Alexander KA, Laver PN, Michel AL, Williams M, van Helden PD, Warren RM, et al. Novel *Mycobacterium tuberculosis* complex pathogen, *M. mungi*. Emerging Infectious Diseases. 2010;**16**:1296-1299. DOI: 10.3201/eid1608.100314

[19] Brosch R, Gordon SV, Marmiesse M, Brodin P, Buchrieser C, Eiglmeier K, et al. A new evolutionary scenario for the *Mycobacterium tuberculosis* complex. Proceedings of the National Academy of Sciences of the United States of America. 2002;**99**:3684-3689. DOI: 10.1073/pnas.052548299

[20] Cayrou C, Turenne C, Behr MA, Drancourt M. Genotyping of *Mycobacterium avium* complex organisms using multispacer sequence typing. Microbiology. 2010;**156**: 687-694. DOI: 10.1099/mic.0.033522-0

[21] Katoch VM, Lavania M, Chauhan DS, Gupta UD. Environmental mycobacteria: Friends and foes. Environmental Biology and Conservation. 2007;**20**(07):87-100

[22] Leclerc MC, Thomas F, Guégan JF. Evidence for phylogenetic inheritance in pathogenicity of *Mycobacterium*. Antonie Van Leeuwenhoek. 2003;**83**: 265-274

[23] Prodinger WM, Eigentler A, Allerberger F, Schonbauer M, Glawischnig W. Infection of red deer, cattle and humans with *Mycobacterium bovis* subsp caprae in Western Austria. Journal of Clinical Microbiology. 2002; **40**:2270-2272

[24] Kubica T, Rusch-Gerdes S, Niemann S. *Mycobacterium bois* subsp *caprae* caused one-third of human *M. bovis*-associated tuberculosis cases reported in Germany between 1999 and 2001. Journal of Clinical Microbiology. 2003;**41**:3070-3077

[25] Arbues A, Lugo-Villarino G, Neyrolles O, Guilhot C, Astarie-Dequeker C. Playing hide-and-seek with host macrophages through the use of mycobacterial cell envelope phthiocerol dimycocerosates and phenolic glycolipids. Frontiers in Cellular and Infection Microbiology. 2014;**4**:173. DOI: 10.3389/fcimb.2014.00173

[26] Jackson M. The mycobacterial cell envelope—Lipids. Cold Spring Harbor Perspectives in Medicine. 2014;**4**(10): a021105. DOI: http://org/10.1101/cshperspect.a021105

[27] Singh P, Rao RN, Reddy JRC, Prasad RBN, Kotturu SK, Ghosh S, et al. PE11, a PE/PPE family protein of *Mycobacterium tuberculosis* is involved in cell wall remodeling and virulence. Scientific

Reports. 2016;**6**:21624. DOI: 10.1038/srep21624

[28] World Organization for Animal Health (OIE). Bovine Tuberculosis Chapter 2.4.6 Bovine Tuberculosis. OIE Terrestrial Manual 2015 [WWW Document]. 2015. Available from: http://www.oie.int/fileadmin/Home/eng/Health_standards/tahm/2.04.06_BOVINE_TB.pdf [Accessed: September 7, 2018]

[29] Pfyffer GE. *Mycobacterium*: General characteristics, laboratory detection, and staining procedures. In: Murray PR, Baron EJ, Landry ML, Jorgensen JH, Pfaller MA, editors. Manual of Clinical Microbiology. 9th ed. Washington DC: American Society for Microbiology Press; 2007. pp. 543-572

[30] Keating LA, Wheeler PR, Mansoor H, Inwald JK, Dale J, Hewinson R, et al. The pyruvate requirement of some members of the *Mycobacterium tuberculosis* complex is due to an inactive pyruvate kinase: Implications for in vivo growth. Molecular Microbiology. 2005; **56**:163-174. DOI: 10.1111/j.1365-2958.2005.04524.x

[31] Giampaglia CMS, Martins MC, Chimara E, Oliveira RS, de Oliveira Vieira GB, Marsico AG, et al. Differentiation of *Mycobacterium tuberculosis* from other mycobacteria with-nitrobenzoic acid using MGIT960. The International Journal of Tuberculosis and Lung Disease. 2007;**11**: 803-807

[32] Nepali S, Ghimire P, Khadka DK, Acharya S. Selective inhibition of *Mycobacterium tuberculosis* by Para-nitrobenzoic acid (PNB) used in Lowenstein-Jensen medium. SAARC Journal of Tuberculosis, Lung Diseases and HIV/AIDS. 2008;**5**:25-28. DOI: 10.3126/saarctb.v5i1.3080

[33] Leisching G, Pietersen R-D, Wiid I, Baker B. Virulence, biochemistry, morphology and host-interacting properties of detergent-free cultured mycobacteria: An update. Tuberculosis. 2016;**100**:53-60. DOI: 10.1016/j.tube.2016.07.002

[34] Niemann S, Richter E, Rüsch-Gerdes S. Differentiation among members of the *Mycobacterium tuberculosis* complex by molecular and biochemical features: Evidence for two pyrazinamide-susceptible subtypes of *M. bovis*. Journal of Clinical Microbiology. 2000;**38**(1):152-157. PMCID: PMC86043. PMID: 10618079

[35] Hayashi D, Takii T, Mukai T, Makino M, Yasuda E, Horita Y, et al. Biochemical characteristics among *Mycobacterium bovis* BCG substrains. FEMS Microbiology Letters. 2010; **306**(2):103-109. DOI: 10.1111/j.1574-6968.2010.01947.x. PMCID: PMC3374e422. PMID: 16704833

[36] Ayele WY, Neill SD, Zinsstg MG, Pavlik I. Bovine tuberculosis: An old disease but a new threat to Africa. The International Journal of Tuberculosis and Lung Disease. 2004;**8**:924-937

[37] McCallan L, McNair J, Skuce R, Branch B. A Review of The Potential Role of Cattle Slurry in The Spread of Bovine Tuberculosis; North Ireland: Agriculture and Food Bioscience Institute; 2014. Available from: https://www.daera-ni.gov.uk/publications/review-potential-role-cattle-slurry-spread-bovine-tuberculosis

[38] Kubica T, Rimma Agzamova R, Abigail Wright A, Galimzhan Rakishev G, Sabine Rüsch-Gerdes S, Stefan Niemann S. *Mycobacterium bovis* isolates with *M. tuberculosis* specific characteristics. Emerging Infectious Diseases. 2006;**12**(5):763-765. DOI: 10.3201/eid1205.050200

[39] Bobadilla-del Valle M, Torres-González P, Cervera-Hernández ME, Martínez-Gamboa A, Crabtree-Ramirez B, Chávez-Mazari B, et al. Trends of *Mycobacterium bovis* isolation and first-line anti-tuberculosis drug susceptibility profile: A fifteen-year laboratory-based surveillance. PLOS Neglected Tropical Diseases. 2015;**309**(9):e0004124. DOI: 10.1371/journal.pntd.0004124

[40] Cosivi OJ, Grange M, Darborn CJ, Raviglione MC, Fujikura D, Cousins D, et al. Zoonotic tuberculosis due to *Mycobacterium bovis* in developing countries. Emerging Infectious Diseases. 1998;**4**:59-70

[41] World Animal Health Organization (OIE). OIE Global Cattle Disease Update. 2018. Available from: https://www.dairyglobal.net/Health/Articles/2018/5/OIE-presents-global-cattle-disease-update-290023E/ [Accessed: October 9, 2018]

[42] Boukary AR, Thys E, Abatih E, Gamatié D, Ango I, Yenikoye A, et al. Bovine tuberculosis prevalence survey on cattle in the rural livestock system of Torodi (Niger). PLoS One. 2011;**6**: e24629. DOI: 10.1371/journal.pone.0024629

[43] World Animal Health Organization (OIE). Zoonotic Tuberculosis Factsheet. 2018. Available from: http://www.who.int/tb/areas-of-work/zoonotic-tb/ZoonoticTBfactsheet2017.pdf?ua=1

[44] Schiller I, Waters WR, Ray Waters W, Vordermeier HM, Jemmi T, Welsh M, et al. Bovine tuberculosis in Europe from the perspective of an officially tuberculosis free country: Trade, surveillance and diagnostics. Veterinary Microbiology. 2011;**151**:153-159. DOI: 10.1016/j.vetmic.2011.02.039

[45] Admassu B, Kebede E, Anmaw Shite A. Review on bovine tuberculosis. European Journal of Biological Sciences. 2015;7:69-185

[46] Johnson L, Dean G, Rhodes S, Hewinson G, Vordermeier M, Wangoo A. Low-dose *Mycobacterium bovis* infection in cattle results in pathology indistinguishable from that of high-dose infection. Tuberculosis (Edinburgh, Scotland). 2007;**87**:71-76. DOI: 10.1016/j.tube.2006.04.002

[47] Thoen CO, Lobue PA, Enarson DA, Kaneene JB, de Kantor IN. Tuberculosis: A re-emerging disease in animals and humans. Veterinaria Italiana. 2009;**45**: 135-181

[48] Deresa B, Conraths FJ, Ameni G. Abattoir-based study on the epidemiology of caprine tuberculosis in Ethiopia using conventional and molecular tools. Acta Veterinaria Scandinavica. 2013;**55**:15

[49] Kuria JKN. Prevalence of tuberculosis is sheep, goats and camel in Kenya (unpublished manuscript)

[50] Sjögren I, Hillerdal O. Bovine tuberculosis in man-reinfection or endogenous exacerbation. Scandinavian Journal of Respiratory Diseases. 1978;**59**: 167-170

[51] Humblet M-F, Boschiroli ML, Saegerman C. Classification of worldwide bovine tuberculosis risk factors in cattle: A stratified approach. Veterinary Research. 2009;**40**:50. DOI: 10.1051/vetres/2009033

[52] Yadav K, Prakash S. Tuberculosis: An airborne disease. Global Journal of Microbiology Research. 2017;**5**:225-243

[53] Flynn JL, Chan J, Lin PL. Macrophages and control of granulomatous inflammation in tuberculosis. Mucosal Immunology. 2011;**4**:271-278. DOI: 10.1038/mi.2011.14

[54] Clemens DL, Horwitz MA. The *Mycobacterium tuberculosis* phagosome interacts with early endosomes and is accessible to exogenously administered transferring. Journal of Experimental Medicine. 1996;**184**:1349-1355

[55] Corrales RM, Molle V, Leiba J, Mourey L, de Chastellier C, Kremer L. Phosphorylation of mycobacterial PcaA inhibits mycolic acid cyclopropanation: Consequences for intracellular survival and for phagosome maturation block. The Journal of Biological Chemistry. 2012;**287**(31):26187-26199. DOI: 10.1074/jbc.M112.373209

[56] Sasindran SJ, Torrelles JB. *Mycobacterium tuberculosis* infection and inflammation: What is beneficial for the host and for the bacterium? Frontiers in Microbiology. 2011;**2**:2. DOI: 10.3389/fmicb.2011.00002

[57] Thoen CO, Kaplan B, Thoen TC, Gilsdorf MJ, Shere JA. Zoonotic tuberculosis: A comprehensive one health approach. Medicina (B Aires). 2016;**76**:159-165

[58] De la Rua-Domenech R. Human *Mycobacterium bovis* infection in the United Kingdom: Incidence, risk, control measures and review of zoonotic aspects of bovine tuberculosis. Tuberculosis. 2006;**86**:77-109

[59] Cezar RDS, Lucena-Silva N, Borges JM, Santana VLA, Pinheiro Junior JW. Detection of *Mycobacterium bovis* in artisanal cheese in the state of Pernambuco, Brazil. International Journal of Mycobacteriology. 2016;**5**: 269-272. DOI: 10.1016/j.ijmyco.2016.04.007

[60] Cousins DV, Huchzermeyer HFKA, Gruffin JFT, Bruckner GK, van Rensburg IBJ, Kriek NPJ. Tuberculosis. In: Coetzer JAW, Tustin RC, editors. Infectious Diseases of Livestock. Goodwood, South Africa: Oxford University Press; 2004;**3**:1973-1993

[61] Ibrahim S, Cadmus SIB, Umoh JU, Ajogi I, Farouk UM, Abubakar UB, et al. Tuberculosis in humans and cattle in Jigawa state, Nigeria: Risk factors analysis. Veterinary Medicine International. 2012. DOI: 10.1155/2012/865924

[62] Une Y, Mori T. Tuberculosis as a zoonosis from a veterinary perspective. Comparative Immunology, Microbiology and Infectious Diseases. 2007;**30**:415-425. DOI: 10.1016/j.cimid.2007.05.002

[63] Grist A. Bovine Meat Inspection: Anatomy, Physiology and Disease Conditions. 2nd ed. United kingdom: Nottingham University Press; 2013

[64] Goodchild AV, Downs SH, Upton P, Wood JL, de la Rua-Domenech R. Specificity of the comparative skin test for bovine tuberculosis in Great Britain. The Veterinary Record. 2015;**177**(10): 258. DOI: 10.1136/vr.102961

[65] Schiller I, Vordermeier HM, Waters WR, Palmer M, Thacker T, Whelan A, et al. Assessment of *Mycobacterium tuberculosis* OmpATb as a novel antigen for the diagnosis of bovine tuberculosis. Clinical and Vaccine Immunology. 2009;**16**:1314-1321. DOI: 10.1128/CVI.00151-09

[66] Clegg TA, Good M, Doyle M, Duignan A, More SJ, Gormley E. The performance of the interferon gamma assay when used as a diagnostic or quality assurance test in *Mycobacterium bovis* infected herds. Preventive Veterinary Medicine. 2017;**140**:116-121. DOI: 10.1016/j.prevetmed.2017.03.007

[67] Liebana E, Johnson L, Gough J, Durr P, Jahans K, Clifton-Hadley R, et al. Pathology of naturally occurring bovine

tuberculosis in England and Wales. The Veterinary Journal. 2008;**176**:354-360

[68] Kuria JKN, Gathogo SM. Concomitant fungal and *Mycobacterium bovis* infections in beef cattle in Kenya. Onderstepoort Journal of Veterinary Research. 2013;**80**(1):585. 4 Pages. DOI: 10.4102/ojvr.v80i1.585

[69] Biet F, Boschiroli ML, Thorel MF, Guilloteau LA. Zoonotic aspects of *Mycobacterium bovis* and *Mycobacterium avium-intracellular* complex, (MAC). Veterinary Research. 2005;(3):411-436

[70] Collins DM. Advances in molecular diagnostics for *Mycobacterium bovis*. Veterinary Microbiology. 2011;**151**:2-7. DOI: 10.1016/j.vetmic.2011.02.019

[71] Oloya J, Kazwala R, Lund A, Opuda-Asibo J, Demelash B, Skjerve E, et al. Characterisation of mycobacteria isolated from slaughter cattle in pastoral regions of Uganda. BMC Microbiology. 2007;7:95. DOI: 10.1186/1471-2180-7-95

[72] Rasolofo Razanamparany V, Quirin R, Rapaoliarijaona A, Rakotoaritahina H, Vololonirina EJ, Rasolonavalona T, et al. Usefulness of restriction fragment length polymorphism and spoligotyping for epidemiological studies of *Mycobacterium bovis* in Madagascar: Description of new genotypes. Veterinary Microbiology. 2006;**114**: 115-122. DOI: 10.1016/j.vetmic.2005.11.057

[73] Haddad N, Masselot M, Durand B. Molecular differentiation of *Mycobacterium bovis* isolates. Review of main techniques and applications. Research in Veterinary Science. 2004;**76**:1-18

[74] Fabrizio V, Giuseppina C, Letizia M, Stefano R, Gesualdo V, Santo C. Detection of *Mycobacterium tuberculosis* complex in cattle by PCR using milk, lymph node aspirates and nasal swabs. Journal of Clinical Microbiology. 1998; **36**(4):1050-1055

[75] Waters WR, Palmer MV, Buddle BM, Vordermeier HM. Bovine tuberculosis vaccine research: Historical perspectives and recent advances. Vaccine. 2012;**30**(16):2611-2622. DOI: 10.1016/j.vaccine.2012.02.018

[76] Farm Crisis Network. Stress and Loss. A Report on the Impact of Bovine TB on Farming Communities. Northampton: Farm Crisis Network; 2009